SPIRITUALITY IN PATIENT CARE

Harold G. Koenig, M.D.

SPIRITUALITY IN PATIENT CARE

Why, How, When, and What

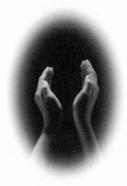

TEMPLETON FOUNDATION PRESS

Philadelphia & London

Templeton Foundation Press
Five Radnor Corporate Center, Suite 120
100 Matsonford Road
Radnor, Pennsylvania 19087

Designed and typeset by Kachergis Book Design,
Pittsboro, North Carolina

Printed by Versa Press, East Peoria, Illinois

LIBRARY OF CONGRESS CATALOGING-IN-PUBLICATION DATA
Koenig, Harold George.
    Spirituality in patient care : why, how, when, and what /
Harold G. Koenig.
        p. cm.
    Includes bibliographical references and index.
    ISBN 1-890151-89-0 (paper : alk. paper)
    1. Medical care.   2. Spirituality.   3. Faith Healing—
methods.   4. Patient Care—methods.   5. Spirituality.   I. Title.
R725.55 .K64 2002   2002018100
615.8/52 21

Printed in the United States of America

03 04 05 06 07   10 9 8 7 6 5 4 3 2

To my daughter, Rebekah Marie Koenig

CONTENTS

SPIRITUALITY IN PATIENT CARE

INTRODUCTION

This book provides a short course for health professionals interested in identifying and addressing the spiritual needs of patients. It is intended as a guide for practicing physicians, medical students, residents, and possibly students in other health professions. The primary audience, however, is physicians who wish to know how to integrate spirituality into clinical practice in an effective, sensitive, and sensible manner. Nurses and chaplains may also find this small book useful as they interact with doctors, other health professionals, and hospital administrators. While several other guides exist on how to address spiritual issues, none of these are readily portable for easy use and rapid access.[1,2,3]

Is there a need for such a guide? Despite the fact that nearly two-thirds of American medical schools in 2001 taught required or elective courses on religion, spirituality, and medicine, few doctors today address the spiritual needs of patients. Even in strongly religious areas of the

United States, less than one-third of physicians even inquire about the patient's religious denomination, and fewer than one in ten routinely take a spiritual history.[4] Many physicians say they feel uncomfortable addressing religious issues or don't have time to do this. Others don't see addressing spiritual issues as part of their job, don't understand why it should be, don't know how or when to do it, and can't imagine what the results would be if they did. This is a book about the why's, how's, when's, and what's of addressing spiritual issues in patient care.

Why? Why address spirituality in patient care? Why identify spiritual needs? Why should this be a routine part of health care? In chapter 1, I examine five reasons why physicians ought to consider this: (1) religious beliefs and spiritual needs are common among medical patients and serve a distinct function; (2) religious beliefs influence medical decision making; (3) there is a relationship between religion and both mental and physical health; (4) many patients would like their doctors to address these issues; and (5) there is a historical precedent for doing so. These five reasons also underscore a need for physician training in this area.

How? How does a physician identify and address spiritual needs? In chapter 2, I describe the process of spiritual assessment, e.g., how to take a spiritual history and instruments for doing so. Next, I examine the role of the physician as orchestrator of resources, supporter of patients' spiritual beliefs, and participant in spiritual activities with patients (such as prayer). I also discuss here the importance of physicians and healthcare systems linking together with religious organizations (through parish nurses or lay leaders) to address the present and future health needs of communities.

When? In chapter 3, I address a number of important issues with regard to *the timing* of spiritual assessment and support. When does one take a spiritual history during the course of medical evaluation—as part of the chief complaint, history of the present illness, family history, social history, physical exam, or wrap-up? Are certain kinds of patients more appropriate than others (for example, a teenager in for a wart removal, a pregnant woman being seen for a prenatal exam, an older person in for a health maintenance visit, or someone being admitted to a hospital, nursing home, or hospice)? How often should a spiritual history be done: once and never repeated, every visit, only at selected times? When does a physician provide spiritual support and what kinds of support are permissible? What about praying with patients? Is this ever acceptable.

What? What results can be expected from addressing patients' spiritual needs? I discuss in chapter 4 the impact that spiritual assessment can have on the patient's ability to cope with illness, on the doctor-patient relationship, patient compliance, and more broadly, on the course of medical illness and response to treatment. Some of the practical benefits of communicating with, referring to, and interacting with clergy in hospital and community settings are illustrated.

Boundaries and Barriers. In chapter 5 I explore limitations in the role that physicians can play in this area. Are there ethical boundaries that should not be crossed? Does medical specialty make a difference? Are there gray areas that must be addressed on a case-by-case basis? What kinds of problems can arise when physicians attempt to address spiritual needs of patients? How can these problems be avoided? Are there other pitfalls and dangers to be aware of when addressing spiritual issues? What are some of the resistances, fears, and concerns of health professionals that prevent them from addressing religious or spiritual issues, and how valid are these concerns?

When Religion Is Harmful. Here I examine the negative effects that religion may exert on health. Are there times when spiritual beliefs can actually interfere with medical care, lead to health problems, or worsen disease outcomes? What are some examples and how often does this occur? How can clinicians handle these cases in a sensitive, thoughtful, and effective manner? Can physician inquiry about spiritual issues cause harm?

Further Resources. In the final chapter, I provide resources that clinicians can turn to for more information about spirituality and health. First, different assessment tools for taking a spiritual history are described and discussed. Second, ten key original research studies on spirituality and mental health, ten on physical health, and ten on social health are presented and briefly summarized. Third, I review academic texts on religion and health, and also summarize popular books on the topic. Finally, websites, newspapers, and popular magazines where health professionals can obtain up-to-date information about spirituality and health are described.

Although this little book will not provide the physician with everything he or she will ever need to know about competently addressing religious or spiritual issues in patient care, it is a good start and will point to key resources to develop further skills in this area.

CHAPTER 1

WHY INCLUDE SPIRITUALITY?

W hy include spirituality in patient care? Why would a physician address spiritual needs or support a patient's religious beliefs? Physicians need to be able to answer these questions clearly and unambiguously before deciding to tackle spiritual issues with patients. Here are five reasons physicians should do so:

- Many patients are religious, and religious beliefs help them to cope.
- Religious beliefs influence medical decisions, especially when patients are seriously ill.
- Religious beliefs and activities are related to better health and quality of life.
- Many patients would like physicians to address their spiritual needs.
- Physicians addressing spiritual needs is not new, but rooted in the long historical relationship between religion, medicine, and healthcare.

MANY PATIENTS ARE RELIGIOUS

Perhaps the best reason for addressing spiritual aspects of illness is that so many of our patients are religious and have spiritual needs. No fewer than 96% of Americans believe in God, over 90% pray, nearly 70% are church members, and over 40% have attended church, synagogue, or temple within the past seven days.[1] Being spiritual, then, is part of who many people are—it forms the root of their identity as human beings and gives life meaning and purpose. Spiritual needs become particularly pressing at times when medical illness threatens life or way of life. In studying 101 psychiatric and medical/surgical inpatients at a Chicago hospital, investigators found that the vast majority of psychiatric patients (88%) and medical/surgical patients (76%) reported three or more spiritual needs during hospitalization.[2] Neglecting the spiritual dimension is just like ignoring a patient's social environment or psychological state, and results in failure to treat the "whole person."[3] Scientists are becoming increasingly aware of the biological pathways by which social and psychological factors influence physical health and susceptibility to disease,[4] and similar influences may soon be identified for spiritual factors as well.[5]

Not only is religion vital to the identities of many people, it is often used to cope with troubling life circumstances—especially sickness and disease. In certain parts of the United States nearly 90% of medical patients report that religious beliefs and practices are important ways that they cope with and make sense of physical illness, and over 40% indicate that religion is *the most important* factor that enables them to cope.[6] According to a Gallup national survey, nearly 80% of Americans say that the statement "I receive a great deal of comfort and support from my religious beliefs" is completely or mostly true (especially persons over age sixty-five, 87% of whom give this response).[7] Religious coping is widespread in patients with heart disease,[8] arthritis,[9] kidney disease,[10] cystic fibrosis,[11] diabetes,[12] cancer,[13] gynecologic cancer,[14] HIV/AIDS,[15] chronic pain,[16] and terminal illness[17] and in nursing home patients[18] and dementia caregivers.[19]

What exactly is "religious coping"? Religious coping is the use of religious beliefs or practices to reduce the emotional distress caused by loss or change. Patients may "turn over" their problems to God, trusting God to handle them so that they don't have to ruminate or worry about them. They may believe that God has a purpose in allowing them to experience pain or suffering, which gives suffering meaning and makes it more bearable. A host of religious cognitions like these are mobilized to reduce anxiety, increase hope, or increase a sense of control. With regard to religious practices that facilitate coping, patients may pray, meditate, read religious Scriptures, attend religious services, perform religious rituals (receive the sacraments or be anointed with oil, for example), or rely on support from clergy or members of their church, synagogue, mosque, or temple. Religious beliefs and practices, then, are used to *regulate emotion* during times of illness, change, and circumstances that are out of patients' personal control.

RELIGIOUS BELIEFS INFLUENCE MEDICAL DECISIONS

Religious beliefs influence the medical decisions patients make when seriously ill. A recent study of 177 consecutive outpatients seen in the pulmonary clinic at the Hospital of the University of Pennsylvania found that nearly half of the patients (45%) indicated that religious beliefs would influence their medical decisions if they became gravely ill.[20] This is a powerful reason physicians ought to know about such beliefs and understand how patients use them to cope.

Religious beliefs can influence the patient's diet both in the hospital and after they are discharged home. They can also influence whether patients will comply with medical treatments, accept blood, vaccinate their children, receive prenatal care, take antibiotics and other prescribed drugs, alter lifestyles, accept referral to a psychologist or psychiatrist, or even come back for medical follow-up.

Religion may influence end-of-life medical decision making, such as a patient's agreeing to a "no code" status or foregoing aggressive therapy in terminal disease.[21] For example, a patient and family may be praying for a miracle in a medically futile situation. That belief could keep hope alive and prevent them from "giving up" (even when giving up is the most appropriate thing to do). Agreeing to a no code status or foregoing aggressive therapy may mean "giving up" to the patient or family. Unless the physician knows about such beliefs, how can he or she adequately manage the patient's care?

RELIGION'S RELATIONSHIP TO HEALTH

During the twentieth century more than twelve hundred studies examined the relationship between religion and health, with the majority finding a significant positive association.[22] Many of these were cross-sectional studies and weak in terms of methodology. There were also, however, many well-designed prospective studies, and even a handful of clinical trials that verified and supported the findings from cross-sectional studies. The results of this research include the following:

Coping and Depression. Hospitalized medically ill patients who rely on religion cope better than those who do not.[23] Patients who depend on religion are less likely to develop depression,[24] and even if they do become depressed, they recover more quickly from depression than do patients who are less religious.[25] This is also true for the caregivers of patients with Alzheimer's disease or cancer, who appeared to adapt more quickly to the caregiver role if more religious.[26]

Many other studies in different populations have identified inverse correlations between religiousness and depression. More than 100 studies examined this relationship during the twentieth century, including twenty-two prospective cohort studies and eight clinical trials.[27] Approximately two-thirds (65%) of observational studies found significantly lower rates of depressive disorder or fewer depressive symptoms in those who were more religious, and 68% of prospective studies found that greater religiousness predicted less depression. Five of the eight clinical trials reported that depressed patients who received religious interventions recovered more quickly than subjects receiving either a secular intervention or no intervention.

Suicide and Substance Abuse. There is even more consensus when rates of suicide and substance abuse are considered. Of 68 studies examining suicide, 84% found lower rates of suicide or more negative attitudes toward it among the more religious. Of the nearly 140 studies that have examined religious involvement and abuse of alcohol or drugs, 90% found a statistically significant inverse correlation between the two.[28] The consistency of findings across these studies is impressive, given that they were carried out in many different populations, by different research groups, and in different areas of the world.

Positive Emotions. Well-being and positive emotions such as joy, hope, and optimism also appear to be disproportionately prevalent among the religious. Of 100 studies in the past century that examined these relationships, 79 found that religious persons had significantly greater well-being, life satisfaction, or happiness than did those who were less religious. Of 16 studies that examined the association between religion and purpose or meaning in life, 15 found that religious persons had significantly greater purpose and meaning in life. Even archenemy of religion Sigmund Freud admitted that "only religion can answer the question of the purpose of life. One can hardly be wrong in concluding that the idea of life having a purpose stands and falls with the religious system."[29]

Social Support. Almost all studies examining religion and social support find a significant correlation (19 of 20 studies). Not only does the religious person have a larger support network, but the quality of that social network is higher and may be more durable than secular sources of support when chronic illness strikes.[30,31]

Physical Health. There is mounting evidence from the field of psychoneuroimmunology that positive emotions and social support are associated with better immune functioning and more robust cardiovascular health, and that the corollary also appears to be true, i.e., that depression and social isolation worsen health and slow recovery from illness.[32] If this is true, and religious involvement is related to greater well-being, more social support, better coping, and less depression, then religious activities may also be associated with better physical health.

Although research examining the relationship between religious involvement and immunity is only in its infancy, several published studies and other unpublished reports suggest a connection. In a study of more than 1,700 randomly sampled community-dwelling older adults, high levels of the cytokine interleukin-6

(IL-6) were significantly more common in those who did not attend religious services than in those who did.[33] High levels of IL-6 are seen in diseases like AIDS and lymphoma and among persons of advanced age, and may be an indicator of a weakened or unstable immune system. Similarly, in a study of 106 HIV-positive homosexual men, those who were more religiously involved had significantly higher CD4+ counts and CD4+ percentages, compared to those who were less religious.[34] Finally, in a study of 112 patients with metastatic breast cancer, women who scored higheron importance of religious expression had significantly higher natural killer cell numbers, T-helper cell counts, and total lymphocytes.[35]

With regard to cardiovascular health, at least 16 studies have examined the relationship between religiousness and blood pressure. Nearly 90% (14 of the 16) reported lower blood pressure among the more religious. This is especially true for diastolic blood pressures,[36] and may help to explain scattered reports of lower stroke rate[37] and lower death rate from coronary artery disease[38] among the more religious.

In fact, there is a consistent relationship between degree of religious involvement and lower mortality in general. Of 52 studies that have examined the relationship between religiousness and mortality, 75% (n=39) found that religiously active persons lived longer than the less religious, 19% (n=10) found no difference, 4% (n=2) reported mixed results (longer or shorter, depending on type of religious activity), and 2% (n=1) found shorter survival among the more religious.[39]

In fact, twelve of the thirteen most recent studies using the best research methodology found longer survival among the more religious. This finding is particularly robust when religiousness is measured in terms of religious community involvement. The difference in survival between those who attend religious services weekly or more and those who do not attend is approximately seven years.[40] Stated differently, religious attendance has the same association with longer survival as not smoking cigarettes does.[41] Bear in mind that most of these studies control for baseline physical health, health behaviors, and social support. Despite this, however, a significant survival advantage continues to be found among the more religious.[42] Religious involvement may also slow the decline in physical functioning that is ordinarily seen with increasing age.[43]

Need for Health Services. Research suggests that religious persons spend less time in the hospital, perhaps because they are healthier and have more support within the community. In a study of 542 patients (age sixty or over) consecutively admitted to Duke University Medical Center, those who attended religious services once a week or more were 56% less likely to have been hospitalized during the previous year (p < .0001).[44] This finding remained significant after controlling for severity of medical illness, level of physical functioning, social support, depressive symptoms, age, sex, race, and education. In terms of actual number of days hospitalized, patients attending religious services at least several times per month were hospitalized an average of six days in the previous year, compared to twelve days for those attending services only a few times per year or not at all.

In the prospective part of the study, patients who indicated they were not affiliated with a religious group were hospitalized at Duke for an average of twenty-five days, compared to only eleven days for persons affiliated with any religious tradition. This large difference in length of stay between affiliated and nonaffiliated patients could not be explained by severity of physical illness, disability level, social support, or depressive symptoms. In fact, when these other variables were controlled, the strength of the relationship between lack of affiliation and longer hospital stay became even stronger.

Implications. There is growing evidence from systematic research that religious beliefs and practices are related to better mental health, better physical health, and less need for health services. This research should help dispel the widespread notion among health professionals that religion is either unrelated to health or tends to worsen it. Nevertheless, many questions remain unanswered. We know that religious or spiritual involvement does not *always* have positive effects on health, and even when it does so, the underlying biological mechanisms are poorly understood. There is a host of new studies now being undertaken at Duke, Johns Hopkins, Harvard, and other leading universities that are utilizing a variety of research methods, from observational designs to randomized clinical trials, to more rigorously test the associations between religion and health.

HOW DO PATIENTS FEEL?

Before physicians begin assessing and addressing spiritual needs, it is important to learn how patients feel about their physicians delving into such a personal area. Do they want this? Numerous surveys, both of the general population and of specific patient groups, have asked this question.

In March of 1996, *USA Weekend* magazine reported the results of a nationwide poll of one thousand adults who were asked whether they believed doctors ought to talk to patients about spiritual faith.[45] Nearly two-thirds (63%) of respondents indicated that doctors should. This opinion increased slightly, to 67%, among older persons (those aged fifty-five to sixty-four). When asked if a doctor had talked to them about their spiritual faith, only one in ten respondents indicated that a doctor had *ever* done so.

In a survey of medical outpatients, investigators surveyed 380 patients receiving care in family medicine clinics located in central Texas and south-central North Carolina.[46] Of those surveyed, 73% believed that patients should share their religious beliefs with doctors. Patients who were more religious were especially likely to want to engage in spiritual discussions with physicians.

Several studies have asked seriously ill, hospitalized patients about their preferences in this regard. The first was reported in 1994 when investigators surveyed 120 patients at Pitt County Memorial Hospital in eastern North Carolina and 83 patients at York Hospital in York, Pennsylvania.[47] The majority of patients (77%) indicated that physicians should consider their patients' spiritual needs, and 37% of patients indicated they wanted physicians to discuss religious issues more often with them. Only 20%, however, indicated that their physicians had ever done so. In a second study published in 1998, a sample of 90 HIV-positive inpatients on the HIV/AIDS floor of the Yale-New Haven Hospital in Connecticut were surveyed about attitudes toward physicians addressing spiritual issues.[48] The majority (53%) believed that it was important for patients to discuss spiritual needs with their physicians. In fact, a remarkable 46% indicated that it would be helpful to have an opportunity to pray with their physicians. (See further discussion about praying with patients in later chapters).

In 1999, researchers surveyed 177 consecutive adult outpatients visiting the pulmonary clinic at the Hospital of the University of Pennsylvania. They asked how patients felt about physicians addressing spiritual or religious issues.[49] Overall, 66% agreed that a physician's inquiry about spiritual or religious beliefs would strengthen trust in the physician, whereas 17% disagreed. Of the 45% of patients who indicated that religious beliefs would influence their medical decisions should they become seriously ill, 94% agreed that physicians should ask patients about religious beliefs. Even 45% of respondents who denied such beliefs thought that physicians should ask patients about them. Only 15% of subjects, however, recalled ever having been asked about spiritual beliefs that might impact their medical care.

In summary, many patients wish their physicians to both know about their religious or spiritual beliefs and address these issues as part of their clinical care. Older adults, those with more serious medical illnesses, and those who are more religious are especially likely to desire this. Remember also, however, that some patients do not wish physicians to inquire about their spiritual or religious beliefs (especially during routine office visits), underscoring the need for sensitivity when addressing these issues.[50] One thing is certain. There is considerable disparity between patient reports of willingness to have spiritual discussions with physicians and patient reports of *ever* having had such a discussion, since physicians seldom address these issues.

HISTORICAL LINK BETWEEN RELIGION AND MEDICINE

While hardly a reason for addressing spiritual issues, it is important to understand the historical link between religion, medicine, and healthcare. Although addressing spiritual needs of patients as part of medical care is seen today as something new and different, this practice is actually a very old one. In fact, only within the past several hundred years have medicine and religion pursued separate paths and physicians ignored these issues. Indeed, throughout most of recorded human history, religion and medicine walked quite closely together. For those wishing a more detailed account of this rich history, the *Handbook of Religion and Health* documents it exhaustively. A brief rendition of the past two thousand years follows.

Prior to the late fourth century, sick people who had no family or friends to take care of them and could not afford private medical care had nowhere to go. There were no "hospitals" as we know them today. That changed in A.D. 370 when Eastern Orthodox Christians established a large hospital for care of the sick in Caesarea (Turkey). The first hospital anywhere in the Western world that provided care for anyone in need, it was built in response to the biblical command in Matthew 25:36–40 to clothe the poor and care for the sick. Over the next twelve hundred years the Christian church built and staffed most of the hospitals throughout Europe and England. Many of the physicians during those years were monks or priests, addressing physical and spiritual needs hand in hand.

During much of this time, the Christian church controlled the major universities where medical training took place and directed the licensing of physicians to practice medicine. In the sixteenth century, the power of the Christian church over medicine began to lessen as the state began to play more and more of a role in teaching and licensure. As the scientific revolution gained momentum in the seventeenth and eighteenth centuries, and the philosophy of the Enlightenment came into being, the church's control and influence waned still further, and by the turn of the nineteenth century, as the French Revolution took place, it all but disappeared. Despite the church's weakening influence, hospitals have remained closely connected with religious institutions up to the present day. By 1950, almost a thousand Catholic hospitals were handling some 16 million patients a year in the United States alone. Today, church-related hospitals, many of which were established around the turn of the twentieth century, care for over a quarter of all hospitalized patients in the United States.

Even closer than the connection between religion and medicine is the historical link between religion and nursing. The profession of nursing came directly out of the church, as the Daughters of Charity of St. Vincent de Paul began to organize Catholic sisters to serve both religious and secular hospitals in 1617. By 1789, there were more than four hundred hospitals run by the Daughters of Charity in France alone. In 1830, a Lutheran pastor started a nursing school in Kaiserwerth, Germany, to train women for a life of service to the sick. These "deaconesses," as they were called, became the Protestant equivalent to the Daughters of Charity. In 1803, the Daughters of Charity officially started the first organized nursing group in the United States at Emmitsburg, Maryland. They modeled their practice after the French, performing both home nursing and institutional care. After receiving "a calling from God" in 1837, Florence Nightingale sought training among the Daughters of Charity and the Protestant deaconesses, later applying the principles she learned to help found the modern practice of nursing.

What about psychiatric care? Given the great divide between psychiatry and religion today, could there ever have been a close relationship between the two? Indeed, there was—and not that long ago. In fact, the first form of psychiatric care in the United States was called "moral treatment,"[51] a system developed at the York retreat in England by the devout Quaker William Tuke. Believing that the common practices of bleeding, purging, and ice baths to treat mental illness would fail to cure patients, he instituted a regimen of compassionate psychological and spiritual treatment based on the idea that insanity was a disruption of both mind and spirit. His success was remarkable, and this form of therapy quickly spread across Europe and then to the United States with the establishment of some of the first mental institutions in Philadelphia, Hartford, and Worchester, which were run by superintendents who were often quite religious. Spiritual care was very much a part of the psychiatric care that patients received in those days; chaplains lived right on the grounds of institutions and held religious services for patients, which the superintendents encouraged.

Among those early superintendents was Samuel Woodward, who in 1844 started the Association of Medical Superintendents of American Institutions for the Insane (later to become the American Psychiatric Association). Not long after that, Woodward (superintendent at the Worchester retreat) and Amariah Brigham (superintendent at the Hartford retreat and also sympathetic to religion) became the founding coeditors of the *American Journal of Insanity* (later renamed the *American Journal of Psychiatry*). Over the next fifty to seventy-five years, however, the positive attitudes toward religion in psychiatry would slowly wane, disappear, and then completely reverse. The final nail on the coffin was placed by Sigmund Freud, who from 1908 till his death in 1939 wrote and spoke widely about the neurotic aspects of religion. His teachings would dramatically change the views of the next generation of psychiatrists toward religion.

SUMMARY AND CONCLUSIONS

Good reasons exist for identifying and addressing the spiritual needs of patients. Many patients are religious and use religious beliefs and practices to cope with illness. Because of this, religious beliefs often influence medical decisions, especially those made when illness is serious or terminal. Many patients would like physicians to address spiritual needs and to support them in this area, especially when the seriousness of illness increases. Furthermore, a growing research database indicates that in the majority of cases, religious beliefs and practices are related to better health and quality of life. Finally, there is a strong historical link between religion and healthcare that has been all but forgotten. Addressing spiritual needs of patients is not new, either in the practice of medicine or in psychiatry. How one goes about doing that in this day and age is the subject of the next chapter.

CHAPTER 2

HOW TO INCLUDE SPIRITUALITY

H ow does a physician include spirituality in patient care? How does one go about identifying and addressing spiritual needs? The following describes the process of spiritual assessment and provides specific recommendations for meeting the spiritual needs that are uncovered. Recommendations include, but are not limited to, listening and showing respect, appropriate referral, supporting the patients' spiritual beliefs, and praying for and with patients. While some of these recommendations are controversial, particularly with regard to prayer, sensible approaches are possible. Finally, this chapter explores how physicians and healthcare systems can link together with religious communities through parish nurses or lay leaders to address the health needs of a community.

THE SPIRITUAL HISTORY

Taking a brief spiritual history is necessary in order to (1) become familiar with the patient's religious beliefs as they relate to decisions about medical care, (2) understand the role that religion plays in coping with the illness or in causing stress, and (3) identify spiritual needs that may require addressing. Taking a spiritual history is a powerful act in itself and serves many purposes, in addition to those just mentioned. First, it sends a message to the patient that this aspect of the person's identity is recognized and respected by the physician. Second, it gathers important information that is useful for understanding the motivation behind many of the patient's behaviors related to health. Third, it provides information about the patient's support system and resources within the community that can help provide care for the patient. Finally, it lets the patient know that this is an area that the physician is willing to discuss in the future, should the need arise.

Chapter 7 describes several instruments for taking a spiritual history. While it is not essential that the physician use one of these instruments, it is important that certain information is collected and done so in a sensitive manner. When choosing an instrument to take a spiritual history, then, there are five qualities that should be considered. First, the questions should be brief and take only a few minutes to administer. Brevity is a practical necessity, given the amount of other information that the physician must gather during an evaluation. Second, the questions making up the instrument must be easy to remember so that important information is not missed. Third, the instrument should be effective in gathering the type of information sought (i.e., have appropriate content). Fourth, the instrument must focus on the patient's beliefs—it must be patient-centered. The information being gathered is about the patient's beliefs and has nothing whatsoever to do with the physician's beliefs. The purpose is to understand the patient's beliefs and what role they play in health and illness, without judgment or attempt to modify those beliefs or lack of belief. Finally, the instrument should have credibility, acknowledged by experts in the field as valid and appropriate.

Even if the clinician has difficulty remembering the exact questions of a particular instrument, there are four basic content areas that should be covered when taking a spiritual history:

• Does the patient use religion or spirituality to help *cope with illness,* or is it a *source of stress,* and how?

• Is the patient a member of a *supportive spiritual community?*

• Does the patient have any *troubling spiritual questions* or concerns?

• Does the patient have any spiritual beliefs that might *influence medical care?*

It doesn't really matter how this information is acquired, as long as the physician collects the information and does so in a sensitive and respectful manner. Delegating these questions to others (the nurse, social worker, or chaplain) is not sufficient. The physician needs to take a spiritual history in order to communicate to the patient that the physician is willing to address these issues as they come up in the future. Furthermore, asking these questions will provide first-hand knowledge of the answers so that the physician can assure that spiritual needs are met and that medical decisions are made in light of them.

NONRELIGIOUS PATIENTS

What does the physician do when a patient indicates at the beginning of the spiritual history that there is no interest in religion and that these factors play no role in coping with illness? As soon as the patient communicates this message to the physician, the spiritual history should take a different tack. Rather than focus on spirituality, the physician might ask about how the patient copes with illness, what gives life meaning and purpose in the setting of the current illness, what cultural beliefs are held that may impact the treatment of the illness, and what social resources are available to provide support at home. In this way, vital information is collected while not offending the patient or making the patient feel uncomfortable or pressured.

BEYOND ASSESSMENT

Taking a spiritual history will provide the clinician with important information about the patient's spirituality and spiritual needs brought on by illness. What does the physician do next? Having identified spiritual needs, what is the role of the physician in addressing those needs? Almost no research has been done to help guide us in determining which actions are more or less appropriate for physicians to engage in, and there remains plenty of controversy on how much the physician should do, other than taking the spiritual history. Sometimes, taking the history is enough; other times, more is needed. The following recommendations are based primarily on clinical experience and common sense.

Orchestrate Resources. If spiritual needs are identified, than a decision must be made about whether the physician is capable of meeting those needs, or whether referral is necessary. Medical professionals will vary greatly in their interest, training, and experience in this area. Regardless, it is the physician's responsibility to ensure that spiritual needs are met by someone, whether the physician is that someone or not. A study of 160 primary care doctors revealed that 69% disagreed with the statement, "Only clergy should address religious issues."[1] Sometimes, relatively simple interventions by the physician can sufficiently resolve an issue. Listening with respect and concern may be all that is needed. Often, however, more extensive help is required, and few physicians have the time or training necessary to address spiritual needs in any depth (even those who are motivated to do so). For that reason, when complicated or complex spiritual issues are present, it is important to refer the patient to experts in this area.

A chaplain who is certified by the Association of Professional Chaplains has gone through extensive training to meet the spiritual needs of patients in medical settings. That training typically involves four years of college, three years of divinity school, and anywhere from one to four years of clinical pastoral education. Formal training is followed by a written and an oral board examination before certification is given. Chaplains are the true experts in this area and should be fully utilized whenever possible. If chaplains are not available, then pastoral counselors or trained clergy from the patient's religious denomination should be consulted.

Some patients, however, refuse to see clergy. Having a long-term relationship with the physician makes the patient feel more comfortable discussing religious worries and doubts with the physician. Sometimes clergy are not available at the critical time when spiritual issues arise, such as in the emergency room or suddenly in the clinic or outpatient department. In such situations, it is important to take a few minutes to address these concerns initially (often simply by listening in a caring and supportive manner), and then later refer the patient for more definitive management.

Other resources that patients may need to meet their spiritual needs are religious reading materials, access to religious services (hospital chapel or television), and time to pray with pastors or members of their church or family. These needs should be honored and the environment adapted so that they can be met. This is particularly true in the hospital setting, where routines often take precedent over patient need, especially in the area of spirituality.

Support Spiritual Beliefs. As the physician takes the spiritual history and learns about how the spiritual beliefs affect the medical illness, it is important to be respectful and supportive. Even if the beliefs are unfamiliar to the physician, are different from what the physician believes, or even conflict with the medical care plan, the purpose is to *enter into the worldview of the patient* in order to understand why the patient believes as she does. (There is further discussion of this topic in chapter 6.)

If religious beliefs are not interfering with medical care and appear to be used by the patient to help her cope, then supporting and possibly even encouraging healthy religious practices may be considered. This step is a bit more aggressive, and some physicians are uncomfortable with doing anything beyond taking a spiritual history, acknowledging and respecting the patient's beliefs, and if necessary, making a referral. Others will feel more comfortable taking this next step. It is appropriate for physicians to support and encourage religious beliefs that bring the patient comfort. Chapter 1 summarizes evidence suggesting that religious beliefs and practices help patients cope better with their illnesses, are associated with less depression, and could affect the course of the medical illness.

The physician may even point out that there is indeed evidence from scientific research suggesting that religious beliefs do help people cope and may affect their health outcomes. Pointing this out to patients who are not religious, however, is probably unwise. Remember that the physician is supporting and encouraging beliefs and practices that are already being engaged in by the patient, not introducing new beliefs or encouraging practices that are foreign.

Keeping support patient-centered is absolutely crucial. The physician is nurturing and encouraging the patient's faith, whatever it is and however much of it there is—at all times being guided by cues from the patient.

Participate in Spiritual Activities. The most controversial aspect of addressing spiritual issues in patient care is whether the physician should himself engage in spiritual activities with the patient, or whether this goes beyond the responsibility and professional role of the physician. The most likely spiritual activity that physicians are to be confronted with is whether or not to pray with patients. There is no controversy if the physician prays silently for patients without their knowledge. Any action beyond that, however, carries with it some risk—risk that some physicians may feel is worth taking and others may not. On the one hand, when a physician prays with a patient, this activity can provide enormous comfort and support and build up the doctor-patient relationship. On the other hand, physician-led prayer can also make the patient feel imposed upon, pressured, and very uncomfortable. Some believe that this activity should never take place between physician and patient,[2] and there are reports of patients' family members actually suing and winning cases against physicians for this activity when done inappropriately (see chapter 5). Others believe that decisions on whether to pray with patients should be made on a case-by-case basis, since appropriateness greatly depends on the patient, the situation, and the physician. (Chapter 3 includes a discussion about when praying with patients might be acceptable and when it is not.) Who initiates such activity may be a key factor.

Patients are more likely to want to pray with physicians than vice versa. In fact, many physicians don't recognize that patients might want this. A study of 160 randomly selected Illinois primary care physicians conducted in the mid-1980s revealed that only about one-third (37%) believed that patients might want to pray with their physicians (this was in reference to older patients with severe or life-threatening medical illness).[3] When patients in the same area were asked if they would like their physicians to pray with them, however, 29% indicated "yes, somewhat" and 53% indicated "yes, very much"; only 5% of patients were definitely opposed.[4] Other studies in medical populations have likewise reported anywhere from 28% to 67% of patients indicating positive attitudes toward prayer with physicians,[5,6,7,8] and 64% of the American populace believes that physicians should join patients in prayer if the patient asks.[9] This is especially true for patients with serious or terminal illnesses, when more than 50% of patients indicate that they would like their doctors to pray with them.[10]

Even in the mid-1980s a significant proportion of primary care physicians reported having prayed with patients. In the study of Illinois physicians mentioned above, one-third indicated that they had prayed with a patient. Of those, only about 10% (6 physicians) reported that the prayer did not help the patient at all, whereas 34% indicated that it had helped "somewhat," and 55% that it helped "a great deal." In a 2001 study of 78 physicians in departments of internal medicine, neurology, surgery, and family medicine at a St. Louis academic medical center, 55% indicated that a patient had requested to pray with them in a non-crisis situation.[11] (If crisis situations had been included, it is likely the figure would have been considerably higher.) Thus, it appears that a significant proportion of patients would appreciate (and might ask their physicians) to pray with them, and that a significant proportion of physicians have prayed with patients, the majority having good results.

There is concern, though, that if a physician says a prayer with a patient out loud in public that there will be an "appearance of religious coercion" (even if the patient requests such a prayer).[12] Ethicists with this belief insist that physician-led prayer is acceptable only if clergy are not readily available. One way to get around this concern is to encourage the patient to say the prayer, while the physician participates by being present and saying "Amen" at the conclusion. Some patients, however, will not be satisfied with this. Others may be so overwhelmed in crisis situations that even though they would want to, they can't pray. Furthermore, some patients may not want to pray with unknown clergy, but prefer to pray with their doctors whom they know and trust.

How does a physician go about praying with a patient? Assuming all of the conditions are met for the appropriateness of prayer as outlined in chapter 3, the prayer should be short, supportive, and comforting, its content consistent with the religious beliefs of the patient. The prayer should probably last less than a minute. Long and complicated prayers said by a physician with a patient in a medical setting are unwise. If the patient believes in a personal God, then it is appropriate to emphasize God's love for that person, asking for peace, comfort, and strength for the patient and the family to help them endure through the illness, and wisdom and skill for the doctor to treat the patient's medical or surgical condition effectively.

There is some controversy about whether or not to pray for divine intervention for physical healing (given the disappointment that may result if physical cure does not result), and it may be best to discuss this with the patient beforehand if there is any question. Many patients appreciate prayer for physical healing. Some physicians may even pray that the medications they prescribe will have a powerful effect, helping the body or mind to heal rapidly and completely. Depending on comfort level, the physician may or may not wish to join hands with the patient or place a hand lightly on the patient's shoulder during the prayer. This also depends on the age and gender of the physician and patient, and again, common sense should rule.

Prescribe Religious Activities. If religious beliefs and practices have an impact on health equivalent to not smoking cigarettes or to physical exercise, should physicians prescribe religious activities?[13] Should doctors urge nonreligious patients to become religious, pray regularly, study religious Scriptures, or attend religious services in order to maintain or improve their health? In most cases, this goes beyond what physicians should do. First of all, religion is a sensitive and deeply personal area of patients' lives, and physicians should not pressure or coerce patient behavior in this area. Furthermore, there is to date no evidence from clinical trials showing that if patients become more religious *only* to be healthier, that this will actually result in better health. Such a prescription would involve an "extrinsic" use of religion to acquire a non-spiritual end, and extrinsic religiosity is not usually correlated with better health. Nevertheless, there will always be gray areas that need to be handled on a case-by-case basis (see chapter 5).

LINKING WITH RELIGIOUS COMMUNITIES

While not all physicians will decide to pray with patients, there are other powerful spiritual strategies by which physicians can help to improve the health of their patients and the quality of care they receive. As healthcare begins to shift more and more into the community and away from costly institutional settings, physicians and healthcare systems need to consider linking with religious communities through "parish nurses" (or lay leaders) to more fully address the health needs of patients and families who care for them. Although this applies to all Americans (70% of whom belong to a church, synagogue, or temple), such linkages are particularly important for meeting the health-education and disease-prevention goals in minority communities, whose populations are often very religious and yet experience high rates of disease and poor disease outcomes. Poor health practices (smoking, alcohol, and drug use), low rates of disease screening (breast, cervical, prostate, and colon cancer; hypertension and diabetes), lack of information about diet, exercise, and weight control, and poor access to healthcare are largely responsible for poor health in these communities. Programs developed within religious communities to address these health issues have been shown to be very effective.[14]

As patients are discharged from the hospital sooner and sooner, increasingly severe and unstable medical problems have to be cared for in the community. Physicians are experiencing more and more difficulty getting patients into the hospital unless they are severely ill, often having to send sick patients home from the office because there is no other place to send them. These trends will increase over the next thirty to forty years as the over-sixty-five population in America increases from the current number of 35 million to in excess of 75 million, when Baby Boomers reach their retirement years beginning around 2011.[15] According to an article written in the highly respected journal *Science*, Ed Schneider (dean of the Andrus Gerontology Center at University of Southern California) indicates that if we simply continue on our current trajectory, then many Baby Boomers will be spending their later years in city parks and on city streets because there will be nowhere to provide care for them.[16]

Religious communities have always been the first to meet the needs of the poor, destitute, and downcast members of society, and they were historically the first to meet the healthcare needs of persons in the community who couldn't afford medical care. Religious communities could be a source of healthy volunteers to provide practical services for sick members and respite for their families. Working with parish nurses (registered nurses who are members of a religious community and provide health leadership there) can help to ensure that the medical plan for a patient is carried out, that worsening illness is identified early, and that appropriate follow-up is obtained. Parish nurses can also mobilize and train volunteers, as well as initiate health education and health screening programs to maintain wellness. Working with religious communities to help meet the healthcare needs of patients after they are discharged back into the community, then, seems beneficial to all. In addition to maintaining open lines of communication with religious communities, physicians can act as consultants to congregational health programs or participate in them by providing lectures and teaching classes.

SUMMARY AND CONCLUSIONS

Addressing the spiritual needs of patients means that physicians must learn to take a spiritual history in a manner that is patient-centered and respectful of the patient's beliefs. A spiritual history provides information relevant to medical care and communicates to the patient that the physician is open to addressing needs in this area. For all but the most simple of spiritual needs that arise during such assessments, referral to chaplains and pastoral counselors should be considered. Physicians may consider supporting and perhaps even encouraging the healthy religious beliefs and activities that patients find helpful. In special circumstances, the physician may consider praying with a patient, although this activity is more controversial and risky than either assessing spiritual needs or supporting the patient's beliefs. Perhaps even more important, lines of communication should be kept open between physicians and religious communities in order to mobilize resources to meet the patient's healthcare needs after discharge from the hospital or clinic. Working with parish nurses and even volunteering time to support congregational health programs are other ways that physicians can meet the physical, psychological, and spiritual needs of patients both within and outside of healthcare settings.

CHAPTER 3

WHEN TO INCLUDE SPIRITUALITY

T*he timing* of spiritual assessment and support is essential in order for the physician to effectively provide comfort, gather necessary information, and send the right message to the patient. When is the best time to take a spiritual history? At what point during the medical assessment should this be done, and why? How often should spiritual assessments be repeated? When should a physician support or encourage the religious beliefs of patients? What about praying with patients? Do certain kinds of patients and situations that call for spiritual assessment and support, and others that do not? Again, no systematic research exists on which to base recommendations, and clinical experience and common sense will once again be our guide.

IMPORTANCE OF TIMING

A patient is in the intensive care unit, coming out of anesthesia following a major life-threatening surgical operation. Another patient is in the coronary care unit recovering from a myocardial infarction. A third patient is in the emergency room immediately following a car accident in which serious injuries have occurred. Raising spiritual issues at these times will probably elicit the same response from each patient above—*fear.* Remember that in the old days (and more recent times as well, in some cultures), when a priest or minister was brought in to see a sick patient, it was to give last rites because death was near.[1] Bringing up spiritual issues at these times, then, may send the wrong message to the patient—that the condition is hopeless and nothing more can be done. Of course, if death is imminent or spiritual issues come up at these times, the physician must be ready to address them.

A healthy patient comes to the doctor's office for the removal of a wart or mole. A patient with a cold comes to see a physician requesting medicine to relieve unpleasant physical symptoms. A woman comes into the hospital ready to deliver her baby. These are not times that it is necessary to bring up spiritual issues (assuming, of course, that the woman about to deliver is not a Jehovah's Witness and will not have a life-threatening hemorrhage during delivery). Each of these patients has a specific agenda for the visit. Such patients do not expect a spiritual assessment and may not appreciate the raising of spiritual issues. Doing so, in fact, may confuse them.

A physician is seeing a patient in the emergency room to sew up a laceration obtained by punching his hand through glass. A physician is covering for one of her partners who is away on vacation, and is seeing the partner's patient for a follow-up exam after hospital discharge. A neurologist sees a patient for Parkinson's disease who is referred by the patient's primary care physician. In most of these situations, the physician and patient have never seen each other before and will probably never see each other again. There is no stable relationship (past or future) between patient and physician, and no real reason for the physician to be aware of the patient's spiritual beliefs.

The timing of spiritual assessment and intervention is crucial.

WHEN TO DO A SPIRITUAL ASSESSMENT

There are specific times when a spiritual assessment is indicated and can be done in such a way that the patient is not surprised, taken off guard, or sent unintended messages, and there is sufficient time to address both medical and spiritual concerns. The best times to take an initial spiritual history are (1) when taking the medical history during a new patient evaluation; (2) when taking the medical history while admitting a patient to the hospital, nursing home, hospice, or palliative care setting; and (3) when doing a health maintenance visit as part of a well-person evaluation.

New Patient Evaluation. When a new patient comes for an initial visit with a physician, a complete history and physical are usually done in the office. Part of the medical history is the social history. The social history usually comes after the past medical history and before the physical exam. It typically consists of asking questions about the patient's job, education, and other members of the family and support system. A brief spiritual assessment fits very nicely at the end of the social history in the section exploring sources of support. Questions about religious denomination, whether the patient is a member of a church, and whether religious beliefs provide comfort or affect medical decisions—all flow quite naturally after inquiring about the patient's family and friends. Information learned from the spiritual assessment should be recorded in the medical record so that it can be referred to when necessary. Doing a spiritual history at this time will not alarm the patient as it might if spiritual issues were raised during more acute medical situations (as above).

Admission to the Hospital. Patients with serious illness requiring hospital admission should also have a spiritual assessment completed during the admitting history and physical, particularly if this has not been done within the past six months, by the admitting physician. Often, however, the admitting physician is not the patient's primary care physician. The hospital may hire specialized physicians called hospitalists to provide the medical care for all hospitalized patients. Since these physicians usually don't have access to the primary care physician's records that contain the spiritual history, they should repeat the spiritual assessment on admission since that information may affect decisions made in the hospital. In case of a surgical admission, the same is true for the surgeon who does the admitting history and will be the main doctor caring for the patient and making medical decisions. If the patient is being admitted for a diagnostic or therapeutic procedure that requires only an overnight stay, a spiritual history is less urgent, although this depends on the kind of procedure being done and for what reason. A spiritual history should also be considered for all patients newly admitted to a nursing home or to a hospice program. Again, this is best done as part of the social history.

Health Maintenance Visit. Many people have yearly physical examinations that focus on disease prevention and health maintenance. More time in the doctor's schedule is usually set aside for a health maintenance visit than for a visit for an acute problem or for a routine follow-up. The physician may ask about different health habits and inquire about the patient's family, job, and life stressors. A spiritual history taken at this time flows nicely after questions about family and stress. Again, raising spiritual issues at this time is less likely to alarm the patient than if brought up when the patient is deathly ill. Regardless of when the spiritual history is taken, medical issues should always be competently and completely addressed before turning to spiritual issues.

REPEATING THE SPIRITUAL HISTORY

Care needs to be taken, particularly in acute hospital settings, so that multiple physicians and other healthcare professionals do not repeat the spiritual history during the same admission. For example, if the primary care physician, hospitalist, surgeon, nurse, and social worker all feel obligated to take a spiritual history, then this will likely overwhelm the patient with repetitive questions. Thus, a good general rule is that whoever is taking primary responsibility for the patient in the hospital should be the person who takes the spiritual history and records it in the medical record. Such notes need not be lengthy, but simply indicate that a spiritual history has been taken, whether or not religion is important to the patient, and how it may influence medical decisions. Nurses, who often do their own spiritual assessments, should be aware if the physician has already completed one and proceed tactfully (and vice versa).

How often should a spiritual history be repeated by the same physician? After a complete spiritual assessment has been conducted and recorded, several years may pass before the spiritual history needs to be reviewed or updated, depending on the patient's health condition. The primary indication for an update is when there is a major change in the person's health, social, or living environment (e.g., onset of a serious illness or accident, loss of a spouse or child, relocation to nursing home, and so forth). Again, admission to the hospital may signal the need to review the spiritual history. In general, common sense and need for information should always dictate the frequency of spiritual assessments.

SUPPORTING AND ENCOURAGING RELIGIOUS ACTIVITIES

Besides taking a spiritual history, the physician may decide to support or encourage the religious beliefs or activities of the patient. Timing here is also important. This is perhaps best done as part of the spiritual assessment when the patient is talking about the role that religion plays in coping. Positive verbal and nonverbal responses by the physician are ways to display support, encouragement, and respect. If the physician learns that religion is important for coping, then this information may be utilized at other times in the future when helping the patient cope with medical problems or life changes.

If the patient expresses current or past interest in religious beliefs and activities, but regrets that such activities are no longer engaged in or cannot be engaged in due to health or transportation problems, then the physician may gently explore with the patient whether she would like to increase involvement in this area and how barriers to this activity might be overcome. Remember, however, it is a fine line to walk when nurturing, supporting, and encouraging religious involvement to avoid inducing guilt or making the patient feel uncomfortable over lack of involvement. The physician must at all times guard against the latter and back off if the patient appears to be responding in a negative manner.

If the patient expresses no interest in religious beliefs or activities, there is probably no room to support or encourage religion.

Instead, the physician may decide to encourage social activities or altruistic activities more generally, without referring to religion or spirituality. Another alternative for the nonreligious patient is to encourage nonreligious meditation in order to elicit the "relaxation response," which has been associated with lower blood pressure, reduced anxiety, and better neuroendocrine and immune functioning.[2]

REFERRING TO CLERGY

If spiritual needs are identified that are not readily addressed by the physician through listening, support, and encouragement, then a chaplain or pastoral referral is necessary. This is particularly true if the patient comes from a different religious background and culture than the physician. Referral may also come sooner than later, depending on the physician's comfort, training, and expertise in this area. Many physicians will be unprepared, feel uncomfortable, and lack the time or interest to address adequately the spiritual needs of patients, and should not feel guilty about referring these patients to those who are true experts. Nevertheless, as noted earlier, the physician cannot delegate all of the responsibility to clergy, and taking a spiritual history is one of those responsibilities that lie solely in the physician's lap. The physician should also attempt to get to know the chaplain staff, which will help the physician learn about their strengths and weaknesses and also acquire information about other pastoral resources in the area.

PRAYING WITH PATIENTS

Praying with patients can be divided into prayer that is physician-initiated and prayer that is patient-initiated. As noted in the last chapter, some experts advise that physicians never initiate spiritual activities with patients, and instead rely on the patient to take the first step. Because of the difference in power status between patient and physician, whenever the physician initiates such activities, an element of coercion enters the picture. This is because the patient may have a difficult time refusing such a request, particularly in this managed care era where patients may not be able to pick their physicians. This is especially true since patient surveys indicate that many patients may not wish to pray with their physicians. For that reason, if physicians decide to initiate spiritual activities like prayer with patients, they should proceed with caution and only if certain conditions are met:

• The physician has the same religious background as the patient (e.g., Christian, Jewish, Buddhist, Muslim, Hindu).

• A thorough spiritual history has been taken so that the physician is *certain* that the patient will appreciate and welcome such an action.

• There is a spiritual need present and the situation calls for prayer.

Physician and patient should have the same religious background. If the physician is from a different religious tradition than the patient, the risk of coercion and undue influence increases (whether intended or not). The content of the prayer is almost always influenced by the religious tradition from which it emerges. For example, praying to God presupposes the existence of a personal God who listens and responds to prayer. While Christians, Jews, and Muslims may have no problem with this, a Buddhist patient might. Furthermore, even among Christians there are disagreements about whether one should pray for divine intervention for physical healing or pray for "God's will" in a situation. Thus, even when religious background is similar, doctrinal differences may influence the content of the prayer. Similar religious background, however, is a relative—not absolute—contraindication to prayer.[3]

A complete spiritual history has been taken so that the physician knows beyond doubt that the patient would appreciate the physician's offer to pray. "Beyond doubt." In other words, the patient is as certain to say "yes" (and to truly appreciate it) as a teenage basketball player would say "yes" to an offer to shoot hoops with Michael Jordan, as certain as a scientist would agree to accept the Nobel prize, as certain as a Virginia resident would take the winning ticket for the state lottery. . . . The point is clear. The physician needs to know the answer to the question before the question is asked. If the patient is heavily depending on religious belief to cope and the physician supports that belief by offering to pray, then this will help reinforce the patient's ability to cope and provide comfort. If the patient is not using religion to cope, then this increases the risk that the physician's offer to pray will be perceived as intrusive and perhaps even upsetting. Unless a thorough spiritual history is taken, the physician cannot know how the patient will react.

There is a spiritual need present and the situation calls for prayer. For most physicians (unless they advertise it as part of their practices), initiating prayer with patients is not something that should be done as a matter of routine. Prayer should be reserved for crisis situations or circumstances where neither the patient nor doctor is in control of the outcome—and the outcome is a serious one (when illness threatens life or way of life). Initiating prayer with patients, if done at all, should not be done lightly.

Even if all three conditions above are met, the physician should continue to remain sensitive and draw cues from the patient throughout the prayer activity. The physician should ensure that the patient feels in control at all times. If these simple basic rules are followed, physician-initiated prayer will almost always be deeply appreciated by patients.

The specialty of the physician may also make a difference in how appropriate it is to initiate a spiritual activity like prayer with patients. A primary care physician who is treating a psychologically healthy and stable patient who is coping with a difficult medical problem may suggest a prayer with less risk than might a psychiatrist who is treating a psychologically frail patient with borderline personality disorder. Although all physicians need to worry about this to some extent, the psychiatrist must be more cautious about broaching boundaries in relationships with patients than does the primary care physician or surgeon. More will be said about boundary issues in chapter 5.

Patient-initiated prayer is less controversial than if the physician initiates prayer, although as noted in the last chapter medical ethicists have concerns about physician-led prayer even when the patient takes the first step.[4] There is certainly less risk of coercion if the patient makes the first move, and to be entirely safe, it may be best to have the patient say the prayer. The physician should sit nearby, perhaps join hands with the patient, and conclude the prayer by saying "Amen."

What about a physician who is an agnostic or atheist? Is it necessary to comply with the patient's request even if the physician doesn't believe in prayer? Is it not dishonest to conceal from the patient the doctor's lack of belief? Again, opinions by experts vary,[5] but it would seem that if a physician can bring comfort to a patient by saying "Amen" ("Let it be so") at the end of a patient-led prayer, then there would be no harm in it—regardless of the physician's personal beliefs. Our calling as physicians is to cure sometimes, relieve often, *comfort always*. If a little child who is sick and afraid asks her doctor to examine her teddy bear to be sure he's okay, would the doctor refuse? No, because he wants to comfort the little girl. Showing kindness and concern for the things that are important to our patients is really what matters here.

SUMMARY AND CONCLUSIONS

Physicians should not conduct a spiritual assessment on an outpatient coming in for a wart removal, a cold, a routine Pap smear, or other minor problem, nor should they conduct such assessments in intensive care settings—unless the situation clearly indicates that spiritual needs are present. Likewise, it is unwise to delve into spiritual matters unless the physician has a long-term relationship with the patient, except in cases where a hospitalist, other specialist, or surgeon is managing the patient's care during a hospital admission and there is limited contact with the primary care physician. The best times for conducting a spiritual assessment include the following:

• When taking the initial history as part of a new patient evaluation

• When the patient is admitted to the hospital for a new problem or exacerbation of an old one

• When the patient is admitted to a nursing home or other chronic institutional setting

• When the patient is admitted to hospice or a palliative care setting

• During a health maintenance visit of a healthy patient

• Whenever medical decisions need to be made that may be influenced by religious beliefs

Having knowledge about the spiritual resources of the patient prior to the sudden worsening or onset of a medical condition is always preferable to having to initiate a spiritual assessment at the time of the acute event (to prevent alarming the patient). The best place in the medical history to take a spiritual history is at the end of the social history.

Spiritual support may be provided during a spiritual assessment and at other times as the situation calls for it. Physicians should feel free to provide simple support for the healthy beliefs and activities that the patient finds helpful in coping with illness, although they should always be ready to refer patients to clergy with experience meeting spiritual needs. Some physicians may decide in carefully defined situations to pray with a patient, either initiating the prayer themselves or agreeing to pray at the patient's request. To minimize risk of coercion, it is safest when the patient initiates and leads the prayer, although this may not always be possible.

Addressing spiritual issues is most important when a serious acute or chronic medical illness is threatening life or quality of life, when a major psychosocial stressor is present that involves loss or change (e.g., divorce, bereavement, sick family member, and so forth), or when the patient is about to undergo a major surgical operation or other procedure where the outcome is uncertain and the patient is having difficulty coping. Time spent addressing spiritual issues, however, should never replace the time necessary to address patients' medical needs comprehensively. If the physician is rushed, though, even a single question asked in a kind and thoughtful manner about how the patient is doing spiritually will convey that the physician cares about what for some sick patients is their central source of meaning and hope.

CHAPTER 4

WHAT MIGHT RESULT?

In practical terms, what might result from physicians' addressing the spiritual needs of patients—taking a spiritual history, supporting and encouraging healthy religious belief, helping meet spiritual needs, and mobilizing spiritual support? What difference could this make in the quality of medical care that patients receive? While there have been no systematic studies examining what happens when physicians address spiritual issues, there is sufficient information to hypothesize the kinds of health effects that might be seen. It could make a difference (either positive or negative) in a range of outcomes relevant to medical practice.

Conducting a spiritual assessment and addressing spiritual needs may affect (1) the patient's ability to cope, (2) the doctor-patient relationship, (3) patient compliance, and (4) the overall course of illness and response to treatment. Communicating with, referring to, and interacting with clergy in hospital and community settings may further influence health outcomes by affecting the quality of support and monitoring that patients receive in their communities. The patient may not be the only one who benefits. From the physician's side, the doctor may experience the satisfaction of treating the whole person and seeing patients happier with their care. Results, however, might not all be positive—and that too must be considered.

ABILITY TO COPE

The effects of belief should not be underestimated. Whether it's religious belief, belief in the doctor, belief in the medical treatment, or any strongly held conviction, belief influences motivations and emotions in powerful ways. This idea underlies the rationale for one of the most common forms of psychotherapy used to treat depression and anxiety in the United States today: cognitive therapy. According to cognitive theory, dysfunctional beliefs and pessimistic thoughts lie at the root of negative emotions such as depression and anxiety. Cognitive therapy seeks to alter dysfunctional beliefs and maladaptive cognitions so that interpretations and views of the world become both more realistic and positive. The rule according to the theory is that positive emotions follow positive beliefs. Religious beliefs are usually rooted in a positive, optimistic worldview.[1] For example, most members of monotheistic religious traditions believe that a benevolent creator rules the universe and responds to human prayer, that all things (even negative events and difficult life situations) have meaning and purpose, and that after death there is hope of eternal life, happiness, and the end of suffering. Such beliefs help people integrate and adapt to negative life circumstances more easily. In particular, they give sick patients hope and help them to persevere in difficult circumstances that are not changing.

If the patient is relying on religious beliefs and practices to cope, then any action by a physician that acknowledges and strengthens those beliefs will likely bolster the patient's ability to cope. Studies tell us that religious beliefs and practices are indeed associated with better coping, less depression, and greater well-being in older adults and those with significant health problems. Religious beliefs predict faster recovery from depression in patients with medical illness. Religious interventions that utilize and support the beliefs of the patient result in more speedy resolution of depression and anxiety. Again, whatever strengthens and affirms the religious beliefs of patients will help them more effectively use those beliefs in adapting to life changes caused by health problems. On the other hand, if religious beliefs or conflicts are causing stress rather than providing support, then helping the patient work through these issues becomes imperative.

How might taking a spiritual history influence the coping process? First, when a physician asks about religious beliefs, religious patients have an opportunity to recount or witness to the doctor how faith has helped them cope. The use of religion as a coping behavior is reinforced by the act of verbalizing the benefits; it makes the person more aware and conscious of those benefits. Second, most patients feel that if a physician asks about something, then it must be important—since doctors don't have much time and they ask only about important things. The fact that religious beliefs and activities are important enough for the doctor to ask about sends a powerful message that further reinforces their effectiveness (and if those beliefs are causing distress, validates the need to ask for help in this area). If the physician also supports and encourages beliefs and practices that provide comfort, then this gives them the "authority" of medical approval, strengthening them even further. As the belief gains power, it has more and more potency to affect adjustment and coping.

In 1910, legendary William Osler (then at Oxford University) wrote a short article in the *British Medical Journal* entitled "The Faith That Heals."[2] In the first sentence, Osler writes, "Nothing in life is more wonderful than faith—the one great moving force which we can neither weigh in the balance nor test in the crucible." Indeed, whatever we as physicians can do to build up the faith of our patients, it is in their best interests to do so.

DOCTOR-PATIENT RELATIONSHIP

The most important component of the doctor-patient relationship is trust. The doctor's recognition and support of a patient's religious belief, as noted above, helps strengthen those beliefs. It also does something else, however. Seeing that the physician recognizes and values what is central to the patient's hope also enables the patient to place greater trust in the doctor. This is especially true for religious patients whose beliefs are so important to their identities. For many patients (more than 40% in some hospital settings; see chapter 1), there is nothing as important in helping them cope as their religious beliefs. These patients put great value and trust in their beliefs because those beliefs have helped them get through difficult situations in the past. If a physician validates the beliefs, this not only empowers the patient but also enables the patient to more fully place his or her trust in the physician and in the medical therapies prescribed. The bond between patient and physician becomes stronger, reinforced by a common belief system about what is important in healing.

We know that if a patient believes in the doctor and believes in the treatment, then the treatment will be more effective. The placebo response is based on the belief of the patient in the treatment. Combine the placebo effect with the actual therapeutic effect, and the effectiveness of treatment is magnified. Although the placebo response has its greatest effect on psychological or emotional states (indeed, it is not uncommon in antidepressant treatment studies to have placebo response rates of more than 40%), placebos also affect the way that physical illnesses respond to treatment. Thus, the patient's belief in the treatment may cause actual physiological changes that move the patient toward recovery.

By asking about the patient's religious beliefs in a respectful manner, the doctor indicates a desire to understand an important part of who that person is. If the physician then supports and encourages those beliefs, the patient's trust in the doctor may be amplified. If the physician goes so far as to actually pray with the patient, then this will confirm even more that the physician can be trusted. In fact, the physician's medical authority may even begin to take on an aspect of spiritual authority. The doctor has now become both physician and priest, capable of fully utilizing not only the power of medical therapies but also the power of the patient's belief and trust. This applies most fully to the religious patient.

COMPLIANCE

We know that compliance is strongly related to a patient's trust in the doctor. In a study of 7,204 adults employed by the Commonwealth of Massachusetts, the physician's whole-person knowledge of the patient and the patient's trust in the physician were the variables most strongly associated with adherence to treatment.[3] With other factors equal, adherence rates were 2.6 times higher among patients whose physicians had whole-person knowledge scores in the 95th percentile compared with the 5th percentile (44.0% adherence vs. 16.8% adherence, P < .001).

Taking a spiritual history and addressing the patient's spiritual concerns can have a positive impact on compliance. First, addressing spiritual issues makes patients (especially religious patients) feel like the doctor is addressing them as whole persons. Consequently, the patient is more satisfied and the physician develops increased credibility in the patient's eyes. As noted previously, not only does the physician now have medical authority but also gains some degree of spiritual authority as the patient places more and more trust in the physician. Greater trust increases the likelihood that the patient will follow the physician's recommendations,[4] such as taking medication as prescribed, making behavioral changes, and complying with other medical therapies. While no study has yet looked at the effects of taking a spiritual history or addressing spiritual needs on patient compliance, research does indicate that religious persons tend to be more compliant with prescribed medication and with keeping doctor visits.[5] Patients who are treated as whole persons, i.e., who have their spiritual needs addressed, will feel more obligated to continue the treatment, even when it takes a lot of effort to comply and the benefits are not yet evident.

Second, if patients feel that the physician understands their religious beliefs or struggles and is receptive to discussing those beliefs, they will be more likely to tell the physician about religious beliefs that conflict with prescribed treatments or use of religious therapies instead of medical treatment. For example, a patient attends a healing service at church and decides to stop all medication because she now believes she is healed. If the physician makes an effort to enter into the spiritual worldview of the patient, the patient will be more likely to trust the physician in this area and share experiences. Having such information will enable the physician to follow the patient more carefully, with full knowledge of what is going on.

MOBILIZING COMMUNITY SUPPORT

Communicating with and referring to clergy in hospital and community settings can influence medical care by affecting the quality of support that patients receive after leaving the physician's office or being discharged from the hospital.

First, if physicians become acquainted with community clergy when clergy are visiting patients in the hospital, they will find that clergy are more likely to support them and the treatments they prescribe. Clergy are also ideally positioned to reinforce the need for regular medical attention. If patients are aware that their clergy know and trust their physicians, then this will help patients do likewise.

Second, the physician's staff (with consent from the patient) may alert the patient's clergy about the patient's healthcare needs after an office visit or discharge from the hospital. This will enable the clergy to mobilize resources in the religious community to provide necessary emotional and spiritual support as well as practical services (e.g., respite services, meals, transportation) for the patient and family.

Third, clergy will be more likely to refer members of the religious congregation to the doctor for healthcare, improving the promptness of attention to medical problems. Physicians who have relationships with community pastors can also influence disease screening and healthy lifestyle practices of church members by encouraging health ministries programs at the congregation level.

COURSE OF ILLNESS

Addressing spiritual issues may impact the overall course of medical or surgical illness and response to treatment. This is accomplished by each of the potential benefits described above: improving the patient's ability to cope, helping the patient work through religious beliefs that create stress, enhancing the doctor-patient relationship, and mobilizing support and disease monitoring at the community level.

First, because of the powerful influence that beliefs have in relieving stress, decreasing depression, and increasing hope, addressing spiritual issues may help to activate or maintain the body's natural systems of healing (endocrine, immune, and circulatory systems). Sick patients who are experiencing a great deal of stress, anxiety, or depression have longer hospital stays and greater mortality.[6] Psychosocial stress has even been shown to slow down the speed of wound healing. It does so by altering the immune-mediated cascade of physiological events necessary for wound closure to take place.[7] Thus, psychosocial stress can prolong recovery after accidents or surgery and perhaps even increase the risk of infection. Anything that improves the patient's ability to cope with illness will reduce anxiety and increase hope, thereby having the potential to improve health outcomes. By supporting religious beliefs that help patients cope with illness and by helping patients work through stressful spiritual problems (usually by referral to trained religious professionals), the physician may be performing important interventions with lasting medical consequences.

Second, treating the whole person by addressing spiritual aspects of illness increases the patient's satisfaction with treatment and trust in the physician. Level of trust, as noted earlier, strongly predicts compliance with treatment. Better adherence to the medical regimen, in turn, will improve disease outcomes.

Third, having greater confidence in the doctor, the patient will have greater belief in the efficacy of treatment that the doctor prescribes magnifying the placebo effect, as discussed earlier. Research has shown that when a patient believes in the treatment, this increases the likelihood that the treatment will be effective (whether the treatment is actually effective or not).[8]

Fourth, by increasing the support that patients receive from their religious communities in terms of spiritual, psychological, social, and practical day-to-day help, this will further improve coping with illness by both patient and family. It will also help to ensure that medical therapies are complied with and prompt medical attention is sought when necessary. Thus, by addressing patients' spiritual issues and beginning a dialogue with community clergy, the physician can both directly and indirectly affect the course of illness.

BENEFITS TO THE PHYSICIAN

Although the primary reason for including spirituality in patient care is for the patient's well-being, physicians themselves may also benefit from addressing the spiritual needs of patients. Because of the demands of both the outpatient clinic and acute hospital setting, there is a temptation for busy physicians to run patients through like cattle—focusing only on their biological needs. As healthcare systems have become more and more concerned with the bottom line, doctors have become more pressured to increase their efficiency at seeing patients. That increased efficiency, however, has come at a cost—a cost not only to patients but to physicians as well.

The fact is that most physicians don't become doctors for the money. If highly intelligent talented young people worked twelve to sixteen hours per day, seven days per week, for seven to ten years to become business professionals, they would earn much more than if they spent that time in medical school and residency. No, most of us become physicians because we want to help people, because we want to make a difference in people's lives and in the world around us. Sometimes, though, medical training and the rigors of clinical practice stamp out that idealism. When that happens, physicians begin to experience emptiness and lack of fulfillment in what they are doing, which may lead them to question their choice of profession.

Physicians who begin to address the spiritual aspects of patients' illnesses sometimes experience an arousal of that buried sense of idealism that drove them to become doctors in the first place. No longer are they simply technicians fixing a physical body like a mechanic fixes a broken-down car. Rather, they become physician-priests in the true sense of the term. As physicians begin to treat their patients as whole persons, they find themselves becoming whole doctors again.

NEGATIVE CONSEQUENCES

This discussion has so far described only the positive consequences of addressing religious or spiritual issues in patient care. Could there also be negative results? Research on the topic, or even any published case reports of negative outcomes from addressing patients' spiritual needs, is lacking, but some sobering stories do exist of what can happen if the physician does not proceed intelligently, gently, and cautiously in this area. Below is a list of negative consequences that could result from addressing spiritual issues:

• A religious patient is offended because the physician is of a different religious background and the spiritual assessment is not tailored to the patient's religious faith.

• The patient's family is not of the same religious background as the physician (or the patient), and is offended by the physician's supporting or engaging in religious activities with the patient.

• A religious patient feels challenged because his religious beliefs are not respected during the spiritual assessment, or because the physician deals with his beliefs in a flippant manner.

• A nonreligious patient is upset because the physician is asking questions that hit a sensitive area in her life; she questions the physician's intentions and resents the implication that she is not religious "enough."

• Bringing up spiritual issues at times of serious illness creates undue anxiety in the patient, as this starts him thinking about whether the illness might be a punishment from God or what might happen to him after he dies.

• An unintended message is sent to the patient that she is nearing death and that nothing more can be done, creating anxiety and causing the patient to lose hope and give up.

• Spiritual issues come up that the physician is unprepared to handle or doesn't have time to address, and there are no clergy readily available to assist.

These concerns often scare physicians away from addressing spiritual issues with patients. As stated earlier, no research has examined how often such negative consequences actually occur; however, overall it appears, both in clinical practice and in research studies, that the positive consequences of addressing spiritual issues far outweigh the negative ones, both in frequency and impact.

The text below reviews four relevant anecdotes reported by

physicians. They underscore the need for caution and sensitivity in this area. (The next two chapters further address issues of professional boundaries and religious harm.)

Recently, a psychiatrist prayed with a patient as part of his work in the Texas state mental health system. It is unclear whether the psychiatrist initiated the prayer or the patient requested it, or whether the psychiatrist took a spiritual history beforehand or obtained consent from the patient. In any event, the prayer apparently confused the patient, who told his family about it. When the family sued, the jury ruled against the psychiatrist and in favor of the family. Sadly, this case caused so much fear locally that it led to a number of psychiatric departments advising staff and residents not to address spiritual issues with patients.

A second case involves a woman whose physician made a diagnosis of metastatic lung cancer. She was very distraught. Her son had also recently been diagnosed with AIDS. Sensing how upset she was, her physician asked if he could say a prayer for her. She said, "Absolutely not," and got up and abruptly left the office. The physician never saw her again. A spiritual history might have helped in this situation by revealing the patient's experiences with and feelings about religion. That may have alerted the physician not to proceed with his offer of prayer (although the patient may have also been upset by the spiritual history). There is a natural tendency for patients to ask "Why me?" when they are in the midst of agonizing circumstances. They may feel angry at God for allowing them to suffer so deeply or for not responding to their prayers. Physicians should display extra caution when approaching such patients with spiritual interventions.

In another case, a Christian physician asked a patient who was a Jehovah's Witness if the patient would like to pray with the physician. The patient said no. When the physician gently explored why this religious patient did not want prayer, she said that the physician's use of the word "God" instead of Jehovah in the prayer would have been offensive to her. Thus, physicians must carefully explore the patient's religious background and find out what kind of a prayer would be most supportive for a given situation.

A fourth case, which occurred in a hospital in Fort Worth, does not involve a physician, but a lesson can be learned from it nonetheless. A medical patient was in the ICU after surgery and had not yet become fully conscious. A social worker at the hospital placed a "tract" (pamphlet encouraging Christian conversion) on the bedside table of the patient. The patient's family, who were Jehovah's Witnesses, saw the pamphlet when visiting the patient. Upset by this, they sued the social worker and the hospital. This case emphasizes the need to always be patient-centered when raising and addressing spiritual issues in medical settings. It is the patient's religious or spiritual beliefs that are to be supported and encouraged, not the beliefs of the doctor or other health professional.

SUMMARY AND CONCLUSIONS

Addressing spiritual issues as part of patient care—assessing spiritual needs, supporting the patient's beliefs, validating religious distress, making appropriate referrals to meet spiritual needs, and in carefully selected cases, even praying with patients—may have a number of potential benefits. It may also have negative consequences for both patient and physician if done incorrectly. On the one hand, it may enhance the patient's ability to cope with illness, improve the doctor-patient relationship, boost compliance with and belief in the treatment, and increase support and monitoring in the community, thereby improving satisfaction with medical care and speeding recovery from illness. From the doctor's side, practicing whole-person medicine may reap deep rewards, leading to greater fulfillment and a return of idealism previously lost. On the other hand, when physicians address spiritual issues without sensitivity, caution, or training, the results can be disastrous—leading to patient and family dissatisfaction and even expensive litigation.

CHAPTER 5

BOUNDARIES AND BARRIERS

This chapter explores the duties of the physician and the limitations in that role as it applies to addressing the spiritual needs of patients. What ethical boundaries should not be crossed? When is informed consent required? Are there gray areas that must be addressed on a case-by-case basis? Are there other pitfalls to avoid and dangers to be alert for when addressing spiritual issues? The following text also explores further some of the resistances, fears, and concerns that physicians have about bringing up religion with patients.

PHYSICIAN'S ROLE

Most jobs have a job description. What about the physician? What are the responsibilities of the doctor? Widely known medical ethicist and practicing physician Edmund Pelligrino has written extensively for more than two decades on the role of the physician.[1] He has developed a model that relies on four words: profession, patient, compassion, and consent. By "profession," he means the obligation to be competent and skillful in practice, the need to place the well-being of patients above self-interest, and the voluntary manner in which physicians offer their skills to the patient who needs them. By "patient," Pelligrino means that the person seeking medical care is suffering and in a vulnerable position, and that the physician has the power to influence the patient's decisions and life. By "compassion," he means that the physician is called to suffer with the patient in sharing the existential situation the patient is in (which suggests a spiritual role as well). By "consent," he emphasizes that the doctor-patient relationship is based on a freely given, informed consent by both parties involved, and that this consent should be made in the absence of pressure or force by one over the other.

In addition to these guidelines for doctor-patient interactions, codes or oaths that physicians often take on graduating from medical school describe what respected physicians historically have believed the role of the physician to be. Among the most famous of these codes are the Hippocratic oath and the oath of Maimonides. Written around the fifth century B.C. by the influential Greek physician Hippocrates, the original oath reads as follows:[2]

> I swear by Apollo the physician, by Aesculapius, Hygeia, and Panacea, and I take to witness all the gods, all the goddesses, to keep according to my ability and my judgment the following oath: To consider dear to me as my parents him who taught me this art; to live in common with him and if necessary to share my goods with him; to look upon his children as my own brothers, to teach them this art if they so desire without fee or written promise; to impart to my sons and the sons of the master who taught me and the disciples who have enrolled themselves and have agreed to the rules of the profession, but to these alone, the precepts and the instruction. I will prescribe regimen for the good of my patients ac-

cording to my ability and my judgment and never do harm to anyone. To please no one will I prescribe a deadly drug, nor give advice which may cause his death. Nor will I give a woman a pessary to procure abortion. But I will preserve the purity of my life and my art. I will not cut for stone, even for patients in whom the disease is manifest; I will leave this operation to be performed by practitioners (specialists in this art). In every house where I come I will enter only for the good of my patients, keeping myself far from all intentional ill-doing and all seduction, and especially from the pleasures of love with women or with men, be they free or slaves. All that may come to my knowledge in the exercise of my profession or outside of my profession or in daily commerce with men, which ought not to be spread abroad, I will keep secret and will never reveal. If I keep this oath faithfully, may I enjoy my life and practice my art, respected by all men and in all times; but if I swerve from it or violate it, may the reverse be my lot.

Allan Butler, a physician from Vineyard Haven, Massachusetts, provides us with this updated version of the Hippocratic oath published in the *New England Journal of Medicine:*

> We physicians shall re-emphasize as basic to our profession the rational ethical principal of minimizing suffering. In the course of our training and practice let us not be so intrigued with the intellectual satisfactions of understanding disease that we forget the priority of this humanitarian principal and the consideration of patients as people. In our role as specialists, let us have empathy with our patients. May we seek the potentialities of physical, mental and *spiritual* [emphasis added] health of each person and family and of society. We shall try new therapy or procedures only in fields in which we are experts and in consultation with other experts and only in which, in the opinion of experts, the possible benefit to the patient outweighs the possible risk. As the effectiveness of our services improves, let us fulfill our mounting responsibility to increase their availability. As the cost of our increasingly effective services rises, let us try to deliver them with increasing efficiency.

Pretense will not enter our practice. Inability to help many of our patients will evoke our humility. Their suffering will be attended with compassion. In our reverence for life, let us not confound our minimization of suffering by compounding it in prolonging life nor give priority to quantity rather than quality of life. In practicing ethical principles beneficial to man, may we do unto others as we would that they do unto us, our children and man's genetic heritage. [3]

Moses Maimonides, who lived from A.D. 1135 to 1204, was perhaps the most important Jewish philosopher of the Middle Ages. Born in the Spanish city of Córdoba, Maimonides fled from southern Spain to Cairo because of rising anti-Semitism in Spain. In Cairo Maimonides worked as a physician, and also became a scholar of Jewish law and a philosopher. He is responsible for composing the following oath that bears his name:

> The eternal Providence has appointed me to watch over the life and health of Thy creatures. May the love for my art actuate me at all time; may neither avarice nor miserliness, nor thirst for glory or for a great reputation engage my mind; for the enemies of truth and philanthropy could easily deceive me and make me forgetful of my lofty aim of doing good to Thy children. May I never see in the patient anything but a fellow creature in pain. Grant me the strength, time and opportunity always to correct what I have acquired, always to extend its domain; for knowledge is immense and the spirit of man can extend indefinitely to enrich itself daily with new requirements. Today he can discover his errors of yesterday and tomorrow he can obtain a new light on what he thinks himself sure of today. Oh, God, Thou has appointed me to watch over the life and death of Thy creatures; here am I ready for my vocation and now I turn unto my calling.[4]

Pelligrino's four words and these oaths emphasize that the responsibilities of a physician go beyond that of a typical employee or of a highly skilled technician. They emphasize that the practice of medicine is more like a sacred, holy calling than anything else and that the duty of the physician is to relieve the suffering of patients with expertise and compassion. They also emphasize that the relationship between doctor and patient is a free one, entered into by mutual consent without coercion, and that the physician is in a position of power over the patient who is vulnerable to the influence of the physician. Butler's version of the Hippocratic oath includes the responsibility of the physician for the health of the whole person—physical, mental, and spiritual. What, then, do these duties of the physician tell us about the limitations of that role and the boundaries that must be observed when addressing the spiritual needs of patients?

ROLE LIMITATIONS

Physicians are limited in their level of expertise. Physicians are not clergypersons, nor are they chaplains who have been trained to help patients resolve complex spiritual problems related to physical or emotional illness. Physicians vary widely in religious background and in knowledge of the religious beliefs and practices of their patients, and many are unfamiliar with religious explanations for illness even in their own religious traditions. Thus, while any physician can take a spiritual history in a respectful manner, learning about the patient's religious beliefs, religious resources, and religious struggles in the face of illness (as a part of a duty to assess the health of the whole patient), most physicians cannot provide theological explanations that adequately meet the spiritual needs of sick patients.

Similarly, any physician can support and encourage the beliefs the patient identifies as helpful and comforting, but few physicians have the expertise to provide advice on what beliefs or practices are most helpful for a particular patient, with a particular illness, in a particular religious belief system. Physicians may even choose to honor the request to pray with a patient, and if specific conditions are met, even initiate a simple prayer in carefully selected cases. However, most physicians do not have the training to advise patients on what to pray for, how to pray, or when or how often to pray, even if asked by patients.

NEED FOR CONSENT

Taking a spiritual history as part of the social history or supporting and encouraging the patient's own religious beliefs does not require detailed discussion and consent beforehand. This is simply part of the comprehensive assessment and support of the whole person that is implied when the patient seeks the physician for medical help. Doing anything beyond simple assessment and support, however, requires the fully informed and uncoerced consent of the patient. Because the patient is in a vulnerable position with respect to the physician, the obtaining of uncoerced consent to a spiritual intervention can be very difficult—not impossible, but difficult. Initiating prayer with patients, for example, should take place only when the physician knows beyond any doubt that the patient would welcome such a suggestion. This is true simply because the patient is not in a position to refuse the physician (who makes critical decisions about medical treatments that will influence the patient's life). Furthermore, the patient doesn't have the power to give consent to allow the physician to provide in-depth spiritual advice or deal with complex spiritual issues unless that physician has the training and expertise to provide such counseling.

The physician also needs to obtain consent from the patient before asking a chaplain or pastoral counselor to see the patient. This is particularly true in hospital settings. Likewise, before discussing a patient's case with the patient's clergy, parish nurse, or member of the patient's religious congregation, the physician must obtain consent from the patient. The patient should fully control and approve any communications between the physician and chaplain, clergy, or others members of the religious community.

BOUNDARIES

Boundaries refer to the limitations in the role of the physician and the limitations in the role of the patient. Boundaries are necessary so that the physician can be as objective as possible when treating the patient and making decisions about treatment. Objectivity is important so that emotional issues do not cloud medical judgments. Boundaries are also necessary from the patient's side to limit the expectations that patients place on their physicians.

Limitations in physician boundaries are more or less set within a given medical specialty, although they do vary across medical specialties. For example, boundaries set for a psychiatrist are narrower than those for a family physician, pediatrician, or surgeon. The reason is that psychiatrists treat patients who are often unsure of their own identity and have difficulty recognizing their boundaries as patients. This is especially true for patients with personality disorders (borderline personality disorder being the most severe). If psychiatrists cross over boundaries, or fail to hold patients accountable for overstepping their boundaries, then the therapeutic relationship may become altered so that effective treatment becomes impossible.

Adherence to relationship boundaries is particularly important when the psychiatrist is performing insight-oriented psychotherapy. The psychiatrist must maintain the tightly defined relationship between patient and therapist so it can be used as a therapeutic tool. "Transference" is the patient's projection onto the therapist of qualities of a significant other, usually a parent. The transference that develops in the course of therapy can be used to help the patient develop insight into and eventually work through habitual problems in relating to others. Counter-transference is the psychiatrist's feelings toward the patient as a result of his own emotional needs and projections, and must be carefully guarded against. Transference and counter-transference issues, then, explain the need for boundaries.

A psychiatrist is in danger of overstepping professional boundaries if he treats the patient in a way that encourages personal friendship or becomes personally involved with the patient or the patient's problems. Such over-involvement threatens to compromise the psychiatrist's objectivity, the development of the transference, and the psychiatrist's ability to use the therapeutic relationship to help the patient. Patients are usually unaware of such boundary issues and so will often test those boundaries by wanting to know more about the psychiatrist, the psychiatrist's family, where they live, and where they go on vacation (as in the popular movie, *What About Bob?* with Bill Murray).

The patient may probe for personal information about the psychiatrist in order to form a personal relationship, but usually in the same maladaptive manner as the patient usually does with other people. It is often that maladaptive way of relating to others that has brought the patient in for treatment. The responsibility of the psychiatrist is to maintain the therapeutic relationship and enforce the boundaries in the relationship by not giving out personal information or fostering personal involvement with the patient. If the therapeutic approach being taken is purely supportive (providing emotional support to the patient), then rigid adherence to boundaries is less crucial—although still necessary to some extent to maintain objectivity.

Boundaries between surgeons and patients are also important to maintain, although to a lesser degree than between psychiatrists and patients. If the surgeon is operating on a good friend, this could increase her stress during the operation. For that reason, the surgeon tries to remain as objective as possible in her feelings toward the patient in order to reduce the risk of surgical error. Boundaries between primary care physician (family physician, pediatrician, or internist) and patient are also necessary, although probably to a lesser degree than either a surgeon or a psychiatrist. Again, when the role of the physician is purely supportive, then boundary issues can be relaxed (but again, not totally dismissed).

Spiritual assessment and support do not typically threaten boundaries between doctor and patient. An exception may be in the psychiatrist doing insight-oriented therapy, where supporting or encouraging religious beliefs would not be proper. Boundaries become more of an issue when a physician decides to pray with a patient or offer spiritual advice. Because religion is such an intensely emotional and deeply personal area (for both patients and physicians), it is more difficult to maintain objectivity after such interventions—not impossible, but more difficult. Again, there is less risk for primary care physicians when dealing with patients in stressful medical circumstances, where providing emotional support is the primary objective. Being aware of the dangers of overinvolvement and making efforts to maintain professional boundaries, however, will help physicians regardless of specialty to increase the therapeutic effectiveness of spiritual interventions.

GRAY AREAS

The importance of knowing one's limits and maintaining professional boundaries cannot be overstated, but we need to keep in mind that there will always be gray areas that must be dealt with on a case-by-case basis. For example, consider the case of an older male patient whom we will call Bill. Bill has several chronic health problems, lives alone, and has become increasingly depressed and socially isolated since his wife died two years ago. Social history uncovers that Bill has no close family members in the area. A spiritual history taken by his primary care physician reveals that Bill is quite religious and used to be very active in his church. Because of a conflict with pastoral staff five years ago, however, he stopped attending services and has not returned. He says that he regrets this and misses the friends he had at church. Sensing that Bill might have a spiritual problem, the physician asks if he would like a referral to see a pastoral counselor. Bill declines, saying that he doesn't want to talk with any clergy. The physician prescribes an antidepressant and provides a referral for secular psychotherapy (which Bill also refuses).

When Bill returns for his follow-up appointment a month later, the physician notes that while his mood has improved, he remains socially withdrawn. At the end of the visit, he asks Bill what happened five years ago when he stopped attending services. With great emotion, the patient recalls the angry discussion he had with the music leader about the type of music played in church. The physician listens attentively for about five minutes. At the end he suggests that Bill consider reconnecting with his former church or finding another one. When the patient returns a month later, his depression is much improved. Bill tells the physician that he has attended church services at his former church for the past two weeks and is reconnecting with many old friends.

In this case, the physician identified a spiritual need by taking a spiritual history. Since the spiritual problem appeared complex, he tried to refer the patient to a religious professional. Seeing the need for socialization, and realizing that the patient would not see a pastoral counselor or any counselor for that matter, the physician decided to address the spiritual problem by gently exploring a little further and then suggesting that he return to church. By taking a few minutes to listen to the patient describe the problem in greater detail, the physician helped him work through it. Addressing the spiritual problem and suggesting a solution went beyond the physician's area of expertise. However, the physician tried the more appropriate route (referral) first, and only when that avenue was blocked, did he decide to take on the problem himself. Furthermore, by suggesting Bill return to attending church services, the physician was not introducing or recommending anything new to Bill, since the spiritual history revealed that this had once been a very important area of his life. While the case had a good outcome because Bill responded well to the spiritual intervention, many other outcomes are also possible.

Real situations are always more complex and complicated than can be addressed by rigidly applying a set of rules. The guidelines presented above, however, provide a framework that will help guide physicians in different situations and maximize positive outcomes.

THE POWER OF CARING

The above text has emphasized the importance of role limitations, the maintenance of relationship boundaries between physician and patient, and the need to be flexible in terms of applying these basic guidelines. This discussion would be incomplete, however, without pointing out that sometimes physicians need to take risks. We often deal with patients who are going through incredibly difficult life circumstances, who are lonely, isolated, and carrying tremendous physical and psychological burdens. They come to us for help, often desperate and with nowhere else to go. Sometimes there is no other way to help them but to get involved in their lives, start to really care as a friend, and communicate that to them. This involves self-sacrifice and going beyond the call of duty, taking a risk that will possibly compromise the physician's objectivity in medical decision making. It is a risk taken out of kindness and compassion. It is a risk that some of the best physicians take all the time.

OTHER PITFALLS AND DANGERS

Most problems that result from addressing spiritual issues occur because the physician either does not follow up on spiritual needs to ensure they are adequately met or steps beyond the boundaries of competency by addressing issues that lie in the expertise of professional religious caregivers. The responsibility of the physician lies in identifying spiritual needs and orchestrating resources to meet those needs. If time is a problem, and delegating that responsibility to others (nurses or social workers) becomes necessary, then the physician must always follow up with the patient to ensure that resources were mobilized to meet the need.

Assuming a patient is religious or has a good relationship with his religious community, without taking an adequate spiritual history, is a pitfall to be avoided. This is particularly true if a spiritual intervention (like referral to a chaplain, discussion with the patient's clergyperson, or initiation of prayer) is considered. Such mistakes are usually made during emergency situations either in the emergency room or the hospital, when there is little time for assessment. The problem is failure to obtain consent due to lack of adequate information. It takes only a moment to check with the patient or a family member about the patient's spiritual orientation and whether a spiritual intervention would be appreciated or best avoided.

Providing spiritual advice to patients is another potential pitfall. When there are similarities in religious background, the physician may be tempted to resolve ideological problems for patients by providing them with correct religious views. This can often deteriorate into religious debates or can overextend the physician into a position that can bring attack or devaluation by the patient. Asking questions to help patients clarify their thinking about the spiritual problem is always better than giving advice.

When addressing spiritual issues, physicians must also be aware of how their own religious beliefs can interfere with their ability to evaluate a situation objectively.[5] For example, a physician with conservative religious views may be tempted to impose those views on a patient seeking an abortion, having premarital sex, or involved in an adulterous relationship outside of marriage or in a homosexual affair. Such behaviors may evoke feelings of disdain or disgust in religious physicians toward such patients, compromising their ability to meet the patients' healthcare needs effectively. In the same way, nonreligious physicians may dismiss the conservative religious views of patients as regressive or Victorian, and allow their personal religious views to influence the quality of care that they deliver. Physicians must constantly be on guard for such "counter-transference" reactions within themselves.

PHYSICIAN BARRIERS

While it is true that doctors must proceed with caution and sensitivity when addressing spiritual issues, many don't even try to do so because of personal resistances, fears, or unjustified concerns about delving into this area. The text above reviewed numerous cautions, pitfalls, and dangers so that physicians will be fully prepared to address spiritual issues in an effective manner, equipped to handle or avoid problems that may come up during the process. This should not, however, frighten anyone away—regardless of specialty—from doing a spiritual assessment and compassionately addressing spiritual issues as they arise. Below are some of the barriers, both real and attitudinal, that keep physicians from assessing spiritual issues in clinical practice.

Lack of Knowledge. Many doctors are not aware of how important religious beliefs and practices are to sick patients, nor do they know about the research that links religious practices to better coping and better health. Because physicians tend to be less religious than their patients,[6] they often don't realize that patients—particularly religious patients—might want them to address spiritual issues or might have religious beliefs that could affect their medical decisions. Finally, most physicians are not aware of the potential benefits of addressing spiritual issues, in terms of the doctor-patient relationship and even the course of the medical illness.

Lack of Training. Although nearly 80 of the 126 medical schools in the United States now have either elective or required courses on religion/spirituality and medicine, most physicians in practice have no training in this regard. Furthermore, the majority of students graduating from medical schools today don't either, as most courses are elective and have small attendance. Many physicians don't know how to take a spiritual history, don't know when to do it, and don't know what to do if spiritual needs come up during the evaluation. Unfortunately, many are also perfectly content practicing medicine exactly as they have been doing and do not wish the additional burden of having to do a spiritual assessment.

Lack of Time. In the late 1990s, a study of 170 Missouri family physicians found that 71% indicated lack of time as a barrier to addressing spiritual issues.[7] Lack of time ranked number one among fourteen barriers that were asked about; lack of training or experience taking a spiritual history was number two (nearly 60%). According to a more recent survey in the same geographic location,[8] however, lack of time was *not* a significant predictor of physicians' addressing spiritual issues. Only 26% indicated that they did not have time to discuss religious issues with patients. Although time is short in the physician-patient encounter, asking a couple of questions about how the patient is doing spiritually does not take much time (less than five minutes and more likely only two or three minutes). If spiritual needs are identified, a referral to a chaplain or pastoral counselor is easily done. Studies have shown that people with emotional problems would rather see a clergyperson than a counselor, psychologist, or a psychiatrist.[9,10]

Discomfort with the Subject. One of the most common reasons physicians do not inquire about spiritual issues is interpersonal discomfort. In a survey of predictors of proactive religious inquiry by physicians,[11] investigators found that interpersonal discomfort (i.e., responding yes to the statement "I am uncomfortable addressing religious issues with patients") was the only independent predictor of physician inquiry. Other significant predictors in the uncontrolled analysis (physician specialty, not relevant to health, not in job description) all lost their significance when interpersonal discomfort was added to the model. Lack of comfort is hardly a good reason to avoid asking about an important area of the patient's life that is so closely linked with physical health and decisions about medical care. As expected in that study, family physicians and internists (primary care physicians) were more likely than neurologists and surgeons to inquire about spiritual issues.

Fear of Imposing Religious Views on Patients. While this is often talked about as a concern, most physicians in at least one study did not agree that this was a good reason for not discussing religious issues with patients. In the Chibnall and Brooks study, 75% of physicians disagreed with the statement "Because physicians may impose their religious views on patients, physicians should not discuss religious issues with them."

Knowledge About Religion not Relevant to Medical Care. In the mid-1980s, the majority of physicians did not believe that religious beliefs or practices of patients had an impact on physical health or medical outcomes.[12] That view, however, is changing. In the Chibnall and Brooks study conducted in 2001, 63% of physicians indicated that patient religiousness affects health. In the same study, 64% of physicians agreed with the statement "Physician acknowledgment and support of patient religious values can improve the process and outcome of healthcare provision"; only 8% disagreed with that statement.

Not in My Job Description. A study of 160 randomly sampled Illinois physicians[13] reported that 69% disagreed with a statement indicating that only clergy should address religious issues. In a study of 115 active members of the Vermont Academy of Family Physicians, the majority believed that the physician has a right (89%) and the responsibility (52%) to inquire about religious factors in patient care.[14] The Chibnall and Brooks study also found that the majority of physicians rejected the notion that addressing religious issues was not in their job description.

OVERCOMING BARRIERS

Lack of knowledge of religion's effects on health and lack of training on how and when to address religious or spiritual issues is easily rectified by training and exposing physicians to research on religion and health. Fear of imposing physicians' religious beliefs on patients does not appear to be a major issue, and the majority of physicians believe that it is both appropriate and the responsibility of physicians to address spiritual issues as part of patient care. What appears to be the major impediment to physician inquiry about religious issues is personal discomfort with the topic. Training and practice in addressing religious issues is the only way to overcome such anxieties.

Inadequate time is still a real barrier to addressing religious issues, despite Chibnall and Brooks's report that only 24% of physicians gave it as an excuse for not doing so. While not every patient needs a spiritual assessment on every visit, it still takes time to find out about a patient's spiritual history and it takes time to be supportive and to address spiritual issues that come up. Physicians may simply have to decide on their own whether this area is important enough to take the extra time when the situation calls for it. As healthcare systems learn about the connection between religion and health, and if future studies demonstrate that addressing spiritual needs improves health outcomes and reduces service use, then perhaps physicians will receive extra time to address these issues, a practice which, in the long run, may result in better care and lower cost. Maybe someday insurers may even reimburse physicians for the extra time they spend with patients addressing spiritual issues—maybe.

SUMMARY AND CONCLUSIONS

It is important to understand the roles and responsibilities of the physician, as well as their limitations as to how far they should go when addressing religious issues. Obtaining patient consent is essential, as is maintaining physician and patient boundaries as they apply to taking a spiritual history, supporting religious beliefs, and praying with patients. Gray areas must be acknowledged in order to prevent a rigid adherence to boundaries and maintain flexibility in these matters. Other pitfalls and dangers of physician inquiry about spiritual issues need to be recognized and avoided. Finally, physicians must examine and overcome concerns and worries about talking about these matters with patients.

CHAPTER 6

WHEN RELIGION IS HARMFUL

What about the negative effects of religion or spirituality on health? Recent articles by psychologist Richard P. Sloan in the *Lancet*[1] and the *New England Journal of Medicine*[2] have challenged the research linking religion and health as weak and inconsistent and have emphasized the harm that can result when the physician addresses spiritual issues. "Do no harm" (from the Hippocratic oath) is perhaps the most important rule in medical ethics. Are there times when religious or spiritual beliefs can actually interfere with medical care, lead to health problems, or worsen disease outcomes? What are some examples and how often does this occur? How can clinicians handle such cases in a sensitive, thoughtful, and effective manner? What about physicians actually causing harm by inquiring about religious or spiritual issues?

NEGATIVE EFFECTS OF RELIGION

Obviously not all of the effects of religion on health are positive, and it is important for physicians to be aware of times when religious or spiritual beliefs may worsen health problems or conflict with appropriate medical care. Throughout history, religion has been used to justify hatred, aggression, and prejudice. Even a cursory examination of world events today will reveal horrible atrocities committed almost daily in the name of religion. Religion can cause people to be judgmental and lead to alienation or exclusion of those not playing "by the rules." Religion may become so rigid and inflexible that it becomes excessively restricting and limiting. Religion may encourage magical thinking as people pray for and expect physical healing as if God were a giant genie at the beck and call of every human whim. If that physical healing does not come immediately, then the person may be disappointed and disheartened, claiming that the prayer was not answered and that God does not care, or worse, that the illness was sent by an angry, vengeful God as a punishment. These uses of religion are common in healthcare settings, causing distress and potentially having a negative impact on illness and its response to medical treatment.

Equally as worrisome, religion may be used *instead of* medical care. Members of certain fundamentalist religious sects may fail to seek prenatal or obstetrical care on religious grounds, greatly increasing the risk of infant and maternal mortality (e.g., Faith Assembly in Indiana).[3] Active resistance against childhood vaccination occurs in a number of religious groups around the world and has resulted in recent outbreaks of polio,[4] rubella,[5] whooping cough,[6] and other infectious diseases.[7] Life-saving treatments may be avoided or discontinued on religious grounds. Patients may stop their medications after attending a healing service in order to "demonstrate their faith." This is done with the best intentions and is completely logical within the particular belief system. Diabetics may stop their insulin, hypothyroid patients their thyroid hormone, asthmatics their bronchodilators, or epileptics their anti-seizure medications. Unfortunately, such decisions are usually followed by negative consequences[8,9] and the physician is left to pick up the pieces (often not knowing why the patient's condition has deteriorated). This is another reason patients need to feel free to talk to their physicians about spiritual matters.

FREQUENCY OF RELIGIOUS CONFLICTS

There are times, then, that religion conflicts with standard medical care and patients decide in favor of religion, rather than risk being alienated from the belief system that gives life purpose, meaning, and hope (and perhaps being ostracized from their social group). But how often does this actually happen? Is this a common occurrence that physicians confront every day in their offices, or is this a relatively rare event that is the exception rather than the rule? Based on what we know from the existing research, conflicts between religion and medical treatments are not very common, but they do occur. When they do occur, however, much attention is generated, ethics committees are convened, newspaper stories appear, and so on. Most of our patients are affiliated with traditional religious groups that maintain sensible policies when it comes to need for medical care, and research suggesting otherwise has often been methodologically unsound.

Consider Asser and Swan's 1998 report[10] in the prestigious journal *Pediatrics* that 172 children died between 1975 and 1995 from parental withholding of medical care on religious grounds. Investigators reported examples of children dying from food aspiration, cancer, pneumonia, meningitis, diabetes, asthma, and other treatable childhood illnesses. The 172 deaths were distributed across twenty-three denominations located in thirty-four states. Careful examination, however, revealed that 83% of the total fatalities came from five religious groups: fifty from Indiana (primarily from Faith Assembly referred to above), sixteen from Pennsylvania (most from Faith Tabernacle), fifteen from Oklahoma and Colorado (mainly from Church of the First Born), five from End Time Ministries in South Dakota, and twenty-eight from members of the Christian Science church nationwide. These are hardly mainstream religious groups, and it is safe to say that the total national membership of all these religious groups combined makes up less than 1% of all Americans.

Furthermore, the methodology of Asser and Swan's study makes it almost impossible to determine how often withholding of medical care from children on religious grounds actually occurs. Even the authors admit that "calculations of overall incidence and mortality rates are not possible in this study as the number of children in the group sampled is not available and the cases were collected in a *non-rigorous manner*" (p. 628). "Non-rigorous" means that most cases were collected over the previous fifteen years from newspaper articles, public documents, trial records, and personal communications obtained from the files of Swan's advocacy group, CHILD. Also, prediction of whether or not these children would have survived with medical care was based on the judgment of a single pediatrician (the study's lead author). The science in this study, then, was largely subjective and the results and conclusions strongly influenced by investigator bias.

There are also conflicts between religion and medicine that affect healthcare in adulthood. Many more examples, although almost no systematic research, exist for religious conflicts stemming from beliefs against receiving blood transfusions (Jehovah's Witnesses), seeking psychotherapy (many fundamentalist Christian groups), or more subtle forms of noncompliance based on religious belief.[11] It is safe to say, though, that a large number of these problems could be avoided or minimized if there was better, more open communication between physicians and patients on spiritual issues.

HANDLING RELIGIOUS CONFLICTS

The key to handling situations where religious beliefs conflict with medical or psychiatric care is for the physician to enter into the worldview of the patient and attempt to understand the logic of the decision. There is always a clear reason in the mind of the patient when health or life is at stake, although this is often hidden from the physician. Unfortunately, the first and most natural response of most physicians is to be offended. The patient has chosen what appears to be a totally irrational treatment instead of the doctor's scientifically proven therapy. This creates anger in the physician and sometimes rejection of the patient in return, leading to arguments and the breakdown of communication.

By entering into the patient's religious worldview, the physician will realize how serious a matter this is for the patient. For example, Jehovah's Witnesses refuse blood products because it is their religious conviction that God (Jehovah) will turn his back on anyone who receives blood transfusions. Rather than risk eternal damnation, Jehovah's Witnesses avoid blood transfusions for themselves and their children. To members of this religious denomination, a few more years spent suffering here on earth is not worth being ostracized from family and friends, and perhaps damnation for eternity after death. Within these patients' worldview, it makes absolutely no sense *not* to refuse blood products. Likewise, patients who attend a prayer service and have emotional experiences that convince them that they are healed pit their faith in God against faith in medicine. And faith in God may mean a lot more to them than faith in the word of the physician.

What is important here is to keep lines of communication open between doctor and patient, regardless of what the patient decides. This may require that the physician accept religious patients' decisions to forego medical care and then medically follow them carefully. As long as patients feel that their beliefs and decisions are respected, they will be much more likely to confide in the physician about these matters and turn back to medical treatments if things aren't working out. Otherwise, patients may feel the need to defend themselves and will delay seeking medical help when they really need it.

In situations where religious beliefs conflict with medical care, sometimes it helps if the physician (after getting consent) speaks with the patient's clergy in order to obtain a better understanding of the patient's decision. This action will help the physician learn more about the religious belief system of the patient, will help to align the physician with the patient's religious authority, and will help clarify any misunderstandings that the patient may have concerning religious beliefs. Patients may sometimes use religious beliefs to justify actions that religious doctrines were never intended to justify. A brief conversation with the patient's clergy can often quickly identify such neurotic or defensive uses of religion and will enable the physician to enroll the clergyperson to help apply pressure on the patient to give them up.

PHYSICIAN INQUIRY CAUSING HARM

Does physician inquiry into religious or spiritual issues actually harm patients? Let's take a closer look at this question.

Upsetting Patients. The argument here is that a spiritual assessment is upsetting to patients either because they don't expect it, because it is too personal, or because they are not religious. Patients come to see doctors to have medical problems addressed, not their spiritual lives assessed. Religion is too personal to talk about in a medical setting, and physicians should not inquire about this area any more than they should inquire about a patient's choice of marital partner (or choice to stay single) or decisions about personal finances. Finally, the patient who is not religious may become upset because physician inquiry about religious issues suggests that they are important and that failure to embrace them is abnormal or pathological.

Patients expect doctors to address issues related to their mental health and physical health. If religious issues had no bearing on either, and had no effect on medical decisions, then indeed inquiry about them would go beyond the professional duty of the physician. Because of the enormous role that religious or spiritual beliefs play in all three of these areas, however, it is important for physicians to address them.

Physicians inquire into many personal aspects of patients' lives because those areas affect the patient's health or medical care. As part of the social history, it is imperative that physicians inquire about the marital status of patients, how many children they have, the kinds of supports they have in the community, and their financial status—which all may be sources of either stress or comfort. Physicians do not devalue patients who are single, without friends, or who are poor, but they do need to know about these conditions because of the potential relationship to health and the kind of support the patients will have once they go back home. Physicians also inquire about and make recommendations concerning many other very private areas in patients' lives *if they are related to health*. This includes genetic counseling for those with genetic disorders who are planning to marry, sexual counseling for those with multiple sexual partners at risk for STDs, and counseling about health habits such as eating, smoking, drinking, and other private behaviors, all of which are deeply personal. Again, because of their relationships to health, they are within the domain of the physician's responsibility.

Physician inquiry about the spiritual beliefs and practices of patients should not offend those without such beliefs if inquiry is done in a sensitive and respectful manner. As noted in chapter 2, if patients indicate that religious or spiritual beliefs are not important in their lives, then the physician should simply go on to explore what other factors provide meaning, purpose, and support. Religion is certainly not the only source of fulfillment for basic existential and psychological needs during illness. Such a transition from a religious focus to a nonreligious one should be done so smoothly and seamlessly that the nonreligious patient hardly notices it.

If the patient has religious conflicts or struggles, they need to be brought out into the open. Otherwise, they may worsen the course of the illness[12] or interfere with medical treatment.

Inducing Guilt. It is common for patients to have existential questions about their illnesses, and most inquire "Why me?" when given a devastating diagnosis. A sick patient may feel that the medical illness is a punishment from God. Again, the logic is not terribly difficult to understand: If devout religious faith is related to better physical health and protection from disease, then illness must result from lack of it. "Linking religious activities and better health outcomes can be harmful to patients, who already must confront age-old folk wisdom that illness is due to their own moral failure."[13]

The fact that questions such as "Why me?" are so common and may affect health outcomes makes it essential that these concerns be brought out and addressed, further justifying physician inquiry. Recent research has shown that patients who feel deserted or punished by God, or who question God's power or love, have an increased likelihood of dying sooner than patients without such feelings.[14] While the physician may not be the best person to address complex spiritual issues like these, someone needs to. As indicated earlier, chaplains and pastoral counselors are trained to address such questions, but need to be alerted to the problem. Many patients with these beliefs, however, are alienated from religion because of their negative feelings toward religion and don't want to speak to clergy, leaving the physician as the choice of last resort.

There is also a risk of inducing patient guilt when physicians inquire about religious or spiritual issues. Physicians take such risks all the time when they inquire about *anything* that is related to health status—whether it is smoking, exercise, diet, or even social support. If a patient has lung cancer, the physician is obligated to ask about smoking even if the question makes the patient feel guilty about having smoked. What physician would not ask about exercise and diet in an obese patient with coronary artery disease, taking the risk of making the patient feel guilty for living a sedentary life or not eating a low-calorie diet?

In fact, all counseling with regard to health maintenance or disease prevention runs the risk of making patients feel guilty if they don't follow recommendations and end up sick. Even recommendations to participate in a support group or social activity can cause guilt in the person who remains reclusive and then develops a recurrence of disease. Does the fear of inducing guilt prevent physicians from addressing these issues or making inquiries? No, it does not, nor should it stop them from doing a spiritual assessment.

There is more to be said, however, about inducing guilt in sick patients for not having enough faith. Even the tiniest amount of intelligence or common sense would demand that physicians not make patients feel bad because they are not religious enough. Physical and mental illnesses have many causes—genetic, developmental, accidental, traumatic—that have nothing whatsoever to do with religion or faith. Even the most devoutly religious people end up dying. Are not all the saints and martyrs now dead? It is often not until a person becomes sick, experiences tragedy, or goes through some period of great suffering that deep religious faith or spirituality emerges out of the struggle. Consequently, those who are the most spiritual often end up being those with the most advanced illness. Thus, it is impossible and often completely faulty to conclude that a patient's poor physical health is due to lack of faith—and physicians should never ever imply this.

SUMMARY AND CONCLUSIONS

Besides the many positive effects that religion may have on health, it can also have negative effects. Religious beliefs cause patients to forego needed medical care, refuse life-saving procedures, and stop necessary medication—choosing faith instead of medicine as their treatment of choice. While this does not occur very often, when it does occur it creates much stir and distress for all involved. Physicians need to learn to respect the decisions that patients make, not become offended or feel rejected. Instead, they need to try to enter into the religious worldview of the patient in order to better understand the logic of the decision. Only in this way can that critical door of communication be kept open between patient and physician. The claim that physician inquiry about religious or spiritual issues can cause harm by upsetting patients or inducing excessive guilt is one that should be taken seriously and prompt physicians to obtain training in this area. Nevertheless, this claim is not so water tight or well-substantiated that it should prevent physicians from addressing an area of vital importance to psychological, social, and physical health.

CHAPTER 7

RESOURCES ON SPIRITUALITY AND HEALTH

This final chapter presents a number of resources to aid physicians in addressing spiritual issues in clinical practice. Included first are tools for taking a spiritual history, which are critiqued based on the five qualities of brevity, content, patient-centeredness, credibility, and ease of memorizing, as discussed in chapter 2. Second are brief summaries of thirty of the best original research studies on spirituality and health, including the top ten studies in each of the areas of mental health, physical health, and social and behavioral health. Third are reviews of major academic texts and popular books that comprehensively address the topic of religion and health. The final section describes websites, newspapers, and popular magazines where health professionals can go to obtain updated information about religion, spirituality, and health.

TAKING A SPIRITUAL HISTORY

Kuhn's Spiritual Inventory. Clifford Kuhn, associate professor and associate chairman of the University of Louisville's department of psychiatry, provides one of the earliest spiritual inventories that taps into seven areas: meaning or purpose, belief and faith, love, forgiveness, prayer, meditation, and worship.[1] Each area is explored with five questions, resulting in a total of thirty-five questions. This instrument probably takes about thirty minutes to administer, and is therefore way too long. However, if one considers only the following five belief and faith questions, it becomes more manageable.

- What things do you believe in or have faith in?
- Has this illness influenced your faith?
- How do you exercise faith in your life?
- How has your faith influenced your behavior during this illness?
- What role does your faith play in regaining your health?

This instrument is relatively brief, elicits considerable content with regard to religious beliefs that influence health, is patient-centered, and has a credible source (published in a peer-reviewed professional journal). It is a bit tedious, however, to remember.

Matthews's Spiritual History. Dale Matthews, an associate professor of medicine at Georgetown University, suggests that physicians ask patients three fundamental questions as part of their initial (intake) evaluation:[2]

- Is religion or spirituality important to you?
- Do your religious or spiritual beliefs influence the way you look at your medical problems and the way you think about your health?

• Would you like me to address your religious or spiritual beliefs and practices with you?

This instrument is brief, easy to remember (I I I = Importance, Influence, Interaction), and elicits good content. The source is a popular book and therefore not as reliable as if published in a medical journal, and the final question is a bit personal, suggesting a more active physician role. Matthews has further shortened this history to just two questions in a more recent peer-reviewed journal publication:[3] "Is your religion (or faith) helpful to you in handling your illness?" and "What can I do to support your faith or religious commitment?"

FICA Spiritual Assessment Tool. Christina Puchalski, assistant professor of medicine at George Washington University Medical Center and director of the George Washington Institute for Spirituality and Health, has developed the following five questions that are easily remembered using the income tax mnemonic FICA:[4]

F - faith	What is your faith tradition?
I - important	How important is your faith to you?
C - church	What is your church or community of faith?
A - apply	How do your religious and spiritual beliefs apply to your health?
A - address	How might we address your spiritual needs?

This instrument is also brief, has reasonably good content, is patient-centered, has been published in a peer-reviewed medical journal, and is easy to remember, meeting all five qualities needed in an assessment tool.

Maugans's SPIRITual History. Todd Maugans, in the Department of Family Medicine at the University of Virginia, Charlottesville, has developed a spiritual history that covers six areas (SPIRIT).[5] The six areas are listed below, with illustrative questions suggested by Maugans.

- **S**piritual belief system
    What is your formal religious affiliation?
    Name or describe your spiritual belief system.

- **P**ersonal spirituality
    Describe the beliefs and practices of your spiritual belief
      system that you personally accept.
    Describe the beliefs and practices you do not accept.
    Do you accept or believe . . . [specific tenet or practice]?
    What does your spirituality/religion mean to you?
    What is the importance of your spirituality/religion in
      your daily life?

- **I**ntegration within a spiritual community
    Do you belong to any spiritual or religious group or
      community?
    What is your position or role?
    What importance does this group have to you?
    Is it a source of support? In what ways?
    Does or could this group provide help in dealing with
      health issues?

- **R**itualized practices and restrictions
    Are there specific practices that you carry out as part of
      your religion/spirituality (e.g., prayer or meditation)?
    Are there certain lifestyle activities or practices that your
      religion/spirituality encourages or forbids? Do you
      comply?
    What significance do these practices and restrictions have
      to you?

Are there specific elements of medical care that you
forbid on the basis of religious/spiritual grounds?

- **I**mplications for medical care

    What aspects of your religion/spirituality would you like
    me to keep in mind as I care for you?

    Would you like to discuss religious or spiritual implica-
    tions of health care?

    What knowledge or understanding would strengthen our
    relationship as physician and patient?

    Are there any barriers to our relationship based on reli-
    gious or spiritual issues?

- **T**erminal events planning

    As we plan for your care near the end of life, how does
    your faith impact on your decisions?

    Are there particular aspects of care that you wish to
    forego or have withheld because of your faith?

This spiritual inventory is perhaps one of the most comprehensive,
hitting on virtually all important content areas. The questions illus-
trate the ways that different parts of the spiritual history can be explored. Of course, such an extensive exploration is likely to take
considerable time, making it necessary to adapt the instrument to
the individual patient. Different clinical situations might prompt
the administration of part of the history at one time and the re-
maining parts at other times. The mnemonic SPIRIT, however,
makes the six basic areas relatively easy to remember. The instrument has been published in a peer-reviewed medical journal.

HOPE Questionnaire. Gowri Anandarajah and Ellen Hight, assistant professors in the Department of Family Medicine at Brown
University, suggest that a spiritual assessment cover four areas that
can be remembered with the mnemonic HOPE.[6] Below is a de-

scription of each of these areas and a couple of sample questions
for each category.

H - Sources of **h**ope, meaning, comfort, strength, peace, love,
and connection.

What are your sources of hope, strength, comfort, and
peace?

What do you hold onto during difficult times?

What sustains you and keeps you going?

O - **O**rganized religion

Are you part of a religious or spiritual community? Does
it help you? How?

What aspects of your religion are helpful and not so
helpful to you?

P - **P**ersonal spirituality and practices

Do you have any personal spiritual beliefs that are
independent of organized religion?

What aspects of your spirituality or spiritual practices do
you find most helpful to you personally?

E - **E**ffects on medical care and end-of-life issues

Has being sick affected your ability to do things that
usually help you spiritually?

As a doctor, is there anything that I can do to help you
access the resources that usually help you?

Are there any specific practices or restrictions I should
know about in providing your medical care?

This assessment tool is relatively brief, easy to remember with the
mnemonic, covers lots of excellent content areas, is patient-
centered (and applicable to patients with different types of spirituality), and has been published in a peer-reviewed journal, again
meeting all five criteria.

ACP Spiritual History. A consensus panel of the American College of Physicians and American Society of Internal Medicine has suggested that the following four simple questions be asked of patients with serious medical illness.[7]

- Is faith (religion, spirituality) important to you in this illness?
- Has faith been important to you at other times in your life?
- Do you have someone to talk to about religious matters?
- Would you like to explore religious matters with someone?

This is one of the strongest of all the spiritual histories, largely because of the credibility of the medical body and journal that are its source. The instrument is brief and easy to remember, although no mnemonic exists to aid memory. It is also patient-centered and does not get too personal by having the physician offer to address the patient's spiritual needs. This tool was published in the *Annals of Internal Medicine* in an article authored by a trio of academic giants (Bernard Lo, a medical ethicist at the University of California at San Francisco; Timothy Quill, a highly respected and widely known physician-author; and James Tulsky, a prominent medical internist and ethicist at Duke). A major weakness, however, is that the questions fail to gather information in several key content areas (identifying spiritual needs, connections with spiritual community, and beliefs affecting medical decision making).

TOP TEN RESEARCH STUDIES ON MENTAL HEALTH

Below is an alphabetical list of the author's selection of the top ten research studies that have examined the relationship between religion and mental health. They were chosen based on an assessment of study design, statistical analyses, and authors' discussion of the findings and integration with other research in the field. A brief summary follows each citation.

- Idler, E. L., and Kasl, S. V. (1997). Religion among disabled and nondisabled elderly persons: Cross-sectional patterns in health practices, social activities, and well-being. *Journal of Gerontology,* 52B: 300–305. **Summary:** Cross-sectional study of 2,812 elders participating in a major Yale epidemiologic study. Religious attendance was positively related to less alcohol use and never having smoked; subjective religiousness related to never having smoked. Religious attendance significantly related to both less depression and greater optimism, but only in subjects who were physically disabled.

- Kendler, K. S., Gardner, C. O., and Prescott, C. A. (1997). Religion, psychopathology, and substance use and abuse: A multimeasure, genetic-epidemiologic study. *American Journal of Psychiatry,* 154: 322–329. **Summary:** Study of 1,902 female twins over five years. Personal religious devotion and depressive symptoms were inversely related; religious measures inversely related to current alcohol use and cigarette smoking; institutional conservatism was inversely related to lifetime risk of major depression. High personal devotion was also associated with less of a response to the depressogenic effects of stressful life events (SLEs) (e.g., there was a significant interaction between religious devotion and SLEs).

- Kennedy, G. J., Kelman, H. R., Thomas, C., and Chen, J. (1996). The relation of religious preference and practice to depressive symptoms among 1,855 older adults. *Journal of Gerontology,* 51B: P301–P308. **Summary:** Prospective study of 1,855 elders (40% Jewish, 47% Catholic) in New York City. Jews were more likely to have mental health visits, take psychotropic drugs, and were 75% more likely to be depressed. Frequent religious attendance was associated with less depression in Catholics, but not Jews; over twenty-four months, Jews were more likely to have emergence of depression. Percentage of persons not attending religious services was significantly greater in both the depression-emerged and the depression-persistent groups.

- Koenig, H. G., Cohen, H. J., Blazer, D. G., Pieper, C., and Meador, K. G., Shelp, F., Goli, V., and DiPasquale, R. (1992). Religious coping and depression in elderly hospitalized medically ill men. *American Journal of Psychiatry,* 149: 1693–1700. **Summary:** Study involving 850 consecutive hospital admissions of men age sixty-five or older. Religious coping was inversely related to self-rated and observer-rated depression, controlling for nine other variables; effects strongest in men with more severe disability. In phase 2, religious coping was the only variable to predict lower depression score on follow-up.

- Koenig, H. G., George, L. K., and Peterson, B. L. (1998). Religiosity and remission from depression in medically ill older patients. *American Journal of Psychiatry,* 155: 536–542. **Summary:** Forty-seven week prospective cohort study of 87 patients with depressive disorder by DSM-III. For every 10-point increase on intrinsic religiosity (IR) scale, there was a statistically significant 70% increase in the speed of depression remission. Among a subgroup of patients whose physical illness was not improving or worsening (n=48), every 10-point increase on IR scale associated with over 100% increase in speed of remission.

- Levin, J. S., Chatters, L. M., and Taylor, R. J. (1995). Religious effects on health status and life satisfaction among black Americans. *Journal of Gerontology: Social Sciences,* 50B: S154-S163. **Summary:** Cross-sectional survey of national probability sample of 1,848 black Americans; split into two equal subsamples for analysis. Using LISREL, religious attendance associated with better health and greater life satisfaction, controlling for age, gender, education, marital status, employment, region, urban/rural, and health; associations significant in both subsamples; subjective religiosity also related to life satisfaction in both subsamples.

- Levin, J. S., Markides, K. S., and Ray, L. A. (1996). Religious attendance and psychological well-being in Mexican Americans: A panel analysis of three generations' data. *The Gerontologist,* 36: 454–463. **Summary:** Eleven-year prospective cohort study of 624 Mexican-Americans from three generations in San Antonio. Religious attendance cross-sectionally correlated with life satisfaction for oldest and middle generations, but not for youngest generation. Baseline religious attendance significantly predicted less depressed mood eleven years later both before and after covariates controlled for the youngest generation.

- Neeleman, J., Halpern, D., Leon, D., and Lewis, G. (1997). Tolerance of suicide, religion and suicide rates: An ecological and individual study in 19 Western countries. *Psychological Medicine,* 27: 1165–1171. **Summary:** Cross-sectional survey of random sample of 28,085 adults. Strength of religious belief associated with less suicide tolerance; suicide tolerance 50% lower for those with religious upbringing, 42% less for Roman Catholics, 84% less for highest quartile of religious belief, and 72% less for highest quartile of church attendance; higher suicide rates in women associated with lower religious belief and less attendance.

- Propst, L. R., Ostrom, R., Watkins, P., Dean, T., and Mashburn, D. (1992). Comparative efficacy of religious and nonreligious cognitive-behavior therapy for the treatment of clinical depression in religious individuals. *Journal of Consulting and Clinical Psychology,* 60: 94–103. **Summary:** Clinical trial examining effectiveness of religion-based psychotherapy (RCT) vs. traditional cognitive therapy (CBT), ordinary pastoral counseling (PCT), and wait-list control (WLC) in the treatment of 59 depressed religious patients. Only RCT condition resulted in significantly lower post-treatment Beck scores than WLC; CBT and PCT had non-significant trend in that direction. Only RCT and PCT showed trends toward lower post-treatment Hamilton scores than WLC. Finally, RCT group demonstrated significantly better SAS and GSI scores (depression scales) than did WLC following treatment.

- Willits, F. K., Crider, D. M. (1988). Religion and well-being: Men and women in the middle years. *Review of Religious Research,* 29: as before 281–294. **Summary:** Thirty-seven-year prospective study of religion and well-being; assessed 2,806 sophomores in 1947 and 1,650 resurveyed in 1984. Church attendance and religious beliefs significantly related to overall life satisfaction and to satisfaction with community (significant after controls). 1984 beliefs and adolescent religious participation (1947) predicted significantly greater job satisfaction (1984) after controls. Concluded that traditional religious beliefs were most consistent correlate of well-being.

TOP TEN RESEARCH STUDIES ON PHYSICAL HEALTH

Below is the author's list of the top ten research studies that have examined relationships between religion and physical health, including studies examining blood pressure, immune function, physical disability, and length of survival.

- Helm, H., Hays, J. C., Flint, E., Koenig, H. G., Blazer, D. G. (2000). Effects of private religious activity on mortality of elderly disabled and nondisabled adults. *Journal of Gerontology* (Medical Sciences),

55A: M400–M405. **Summary:** Six-year prospective study of 3,768 older adults in North Carolina. Private religious activity (meditation, prayer, or Bible study) related to mortality in healthy but not disabled subjects; persons with no disability and little or no private religious activity in 1986 were significantly more likely to die during the follow-up (47% more likely), after multiple controls for health, social support, and health behaviors.

- Hummer, R., Rogers, R., Nam, C., and Ellison, C. G. (1999). Religious involvement and U.S. adult mortality. *Demography,* 36: 273–285. **Summary:** Nine-year prospective study of national sample of 21,204 adults of all ages. Nonattenders at religious services lived to average age of fifty-five years beyond age twenty, compared with sixty-two years for those attending weekly or more (seven-year difference); among blacks, life expectancy beyond age twenty for more than weekly attenders was sixty years, compared with forty-six years for those never attending church (fourteen-year difference).

- Goldbourt, U., Yaari, S., and Medalie, J. H. (1993). Factors predictive of long-term coronary heart disease mortality among 10,059 male Israeli civil servants and municipal employees. *Cardiology,* 82: 100–121. **Summary:** Twenty-three-year prospective study of 10,059 Jewish male civil servants aged forty or over in Israel. Religious orthodoxy related to lower mortality from coronary artery disease (CAD); the risk of death from CAD among most orthodox believers 20% less; results remained significant after controlling for age, blood pressure, cholesterol, smoking, diabetes, body mass index, and baseline coronary artery disease.

- Idler, E. L., and Kasl, S. V. (1997). Religion among disabled and nondisabled elderly persons, II: Attendance at religious services as a predictor of the course of disability. *Journal of Gerontology,* 52B:

S306–S316. **Summary:** Twelve-year prospective study of 2,812 elders in Yale EPESE; frequent 1982 attendance predicted lower disability throughout the follow-up period (controlled for twenty covariates); 1982 functional disability, however, did not have long-term effect in preventing church attendance during follow-up. Attendance may delay onset of disability, an effect that is greater than disability's effect on preventing attendance.

- Koenig, H. G., Hays, J. C., Larson, D. B., George, L. K., Cohen, H. J., McCullough, M., Meador, K., Blazer, D. G. (1999). Does religious attendance prolong survival?: A six-year follow-up study of 3,968 older adults. *Journal of Gerontology* (Medical Sciences), 54A: M370–M377. **Summary:** 3,968 adults ages 64-101 years in North Carolina. During median 6.3 year follow-up, relative hazard (RH) of dying for frequent attenders was 46% less; effect strongest in women (49% less) but also present in men (37% less); controlling for multiple covariates, effect weakened but remained significant for entire sample (28% less), both women (35% less) and men (27% less).

- Pargament, K. I., Koenig, H. G., Tarakeshwar, N., Hahn, J. (2001, August 13). Religious struggle as a predictor of mortality among medically ill elderly patients: A two-year longitudinal study. *Archives of Internal Medicine* 161: 1881–1885. **Summary:** Two-year prospective study of 595 hospitalized patients; characteristics of 268 survivors compared with those of deceased patients. Religious struggle (feeling abandoned or punished by God, questioning God's love and power, feeling abandoned by church, feeling devil caused health problems) associated with increased risk of death (6% higher for every 1-point increase on 21-point religious struggle scale, controlling for demographics, physical and mental health, and social support).

- Schneider, R. H., Staggers, F., Alexander, C., Sheppard, W., Rainforth, M., Kondwani, K., Smith, S., and King, C. G. (1995). A randomized, controlled trial of stress reduction for hypertension in older African Americans. *Hypertension,* 26: 820–829. **Summary:** 111 African Americans in Oakland, CA, ages fifty-five to eighty-five, with mild hypertension; randomized, controlled single-blind trial of Transcendental Meditation (TM) compared with progressive muscle relaxation (PMR) and life-style modification (LSM). TM had significantly greater effects on blood pressure (BP) than did PMR; TM was twice as effective as PMR in reducing systolic and diastolic BP.

- Strawbridge, W. J., Cohen, R. D., Shema, S. J., and Kaplan, G. A. (1997). Frequent attendance at religious services and mortality over twenty-eight years. *American Journal of Public Health,* 87: 957 –961. **Summary:** Twenty-eight-year prospective study of 5,286 Alameda County residents of all ages. Likelihood of dying for weekly attenders at religious services in 1965 was 36% less during follow-up; adjusting for social and health practices reduced effect to 23% (still highly significant). During follow-up, frequent attenders more likely to stop smoking, increase exercising, increase social contacts, and stay married, yet these factors were still unable to explain mortality effect.

- Timio, M., Verdecchia, P., Venanzi, S., Gentili, S., Ronconi, M., Francucci, B., Montanari, M., and Bichisao, E. (1988). Age and blood pressure changes. A 20-year follow-up study in nuns in a secluded order. *Hypertension,* 12: 457–461. **Summary:** Twenty-year prospective study of 144 nuns in a monastic order and 138 laywomen controls. While average blood pressures (BP) in the two groups was equal at start of study, BP increased over time only in laywomen (p < .0001), adjusting for education, race, weight, body mass index, smoking, family history of hypertension, serum cholesterol and triglycerides, and twenty-four-hour urinary sodium excretion.

- Woods, T. E., Antoni, M. H., Ironson, G. H., and Kling, D. W. (1999). Religiosity is associated with affective and immune status in symptomatic HIV-infected gay men. *Journal of Psychosomatic Research,* 46: 165–176. **Summary:** Study of 106 HIV+ gay men. Religious activities (prayer, religious attendance, spiritual discussions, reading religious/spiritual literature) associated with significantly higher CD4+ counts and CD4+ percentages; effects on immune function not confounded by disease progression. Religious coping related to less depression and lower anxiety.

TOP TEN RESEARCH STUDIES ON SOCIAL HEALTH

Below is the author's list of the top ten research studies that have examined relationships between religion and social and behavioral health, including miscellaneous factors such as social support, health behaviors, substance abuse, marital stability, and sexual practices.

- Amey, C. H., Albrecht, S. L., and Miller, M. K. (1996). Racial differences in adolescent drug use: The impact of religion. *Substance Use and Misuse,* 31: 1311–1332. **Summary:** National survey of 11,728 high school seniors in 130 high schools. Religious involvement (affiliation, importance, and attendance) was inversely related to use of cigarettes, alcohol, marijuana, and other drugs; significant interactions found for race suggesting that religion is more of a deterrent for drug use among whites than among blacks.

- Bradley, D. E. (1995). Religious involvement and social resources: Evidence from the data set, "Americans' Changing Lives". *Journal for the Scientific Study of Religion,* 34: 259–267. **Summary:** National sample of 3,597 adults. Church attendance strongly correlated with support network size, in-person contacts, and perceived quality of relationships; frequent attenders on average had three more persons to call on for help than infrequent attenders, 13% more telephone contacts, and 9% more in-person contacts. Concluded attendance associated with larger, denser social networks, and more exchanges of goods, services, and information.

- Call, V. R. A., and Heaton, T. B. (1997). Religious influence on marital stability. *Journal for the Scientific Study of Religion,* 36: 382–392. **Summary:** National survey of 4,587 couples to determine relationship between religiosity and marital stability. Persons with no affiliation and mixed marriages had the greatest likelihood of divorce/separation; the wife's frequency of religious attendance, the difference between wife's and husband's religious attendance, and the wife's strength of religious belief predicted a lower likelihood of separation/divorce.

- Cochran, J. K., and Beeghley, L. (1991). The influence of religion on attitudes toward nonmarital sexuality: A preliminary assessment of reference group theory. *Journal for the Scientific Study of Religion,* 30: 45–62. **Summary:** National sample of 14,979 adults in U.S. surveyed concerning premarital and extramarital sex. Church attendance, strength of religious beliefs, belief in afterlife, and church membership all inversely related to permissive attitudes toward premarital sex (after multiple controls); for extramarital sex, all were inversely related to permissive attitudes except church membership. Effects strongest among Baptists and non-mainline Protestants, and weakest among Jews and those with no affiliation.

- Ellison, C. G., and George, L. K. (1994). Religious involvement, social ties, and social support in a southeastern community. *Journal for the Scientific Study of Religion,* 33: 46–61. **Summary:** Survey of 2,956 persons in NC Piedmont site of the NIMH Epidemiologic Catchment Area. Church attendance significantly related to non-kin ties, in-person contacts, and telephone calls, as well as received instrumental support. There was also a significant relationship between church attendance and quality of social support.

- Hatch, L. R. (1991). Informal support patterns of older African American and white women. *Research on Aging,* 13: 144–170. **Summary:** National survey of 1,439 women age sixty or over; examined whom subjects would call on to provide help in terms of an emergency, to borrow $200, or for help or advice when feeling depressed or confused. Help received from non-relatives was significantly associated with participation in religious social events; greater participation also associated with more help given to non-relatives. Greater involvement in religious activities associated with greater help given to and provided by non-relatives.

- Koenig, H. G., George, L. K., Cohen, H. J., Hays, J. C., Blazer, D. G., Larson, D. B. (1998). The relationship between religious activities and cigarette smoking in older adults. *Journal of Gerontology, Medical Sciences,* 53A: M426–M434. **Summary:** Study of 3,968 persons age sixty-five years or older in three-wave EPESE survey. Frequent religious attenders were significantly less likely to smoke cigarettes (present at all three waves); private religious activity at least daily was associated with less smoking (waves 2 and 3). Those who both attended services weekly or more *and* prayed/studied Bible daily (n=1329) were almost 90% more likely not to smoke.

- Koenig, H. G., George, L. K., Meador, K. G., Blazer, D. G., and Ford, S. M. (1994). The relationship between religion and alcoholism in a sample of community-dwelling adults. *Hospital and Community Psychiatry,* 45: 225–231. **Summary:** Cross-sectional study of 2,969 participants ages eighteen to ninety-seven in North Carolina; outcome was six month and lifetime DSM-III alcohol abuse/dependence (AAD). Persons who prayed/read Bible several times/week were 58% less likely to have AAD in past six months after controlling for age, sex, race, SES, and health status; frequent religious attenders were 71% less likely in past six months and 52% less likely in lifetime; "born again" people 39% less likely in past six months and 32% less likely in lifetime.

- Seidman, S. N., Mosher, W. D., and Aral, S. O. (1992). Women with multiple sexual partners: United States, 1988. *American Journal of Public Health,* 82: 1388–1394. **Summary:** National survey of 7,011 sexually active women ages fifteen to forty-four. Those with a religious affiliation were less likely than those without to have multiple sexual partners (3.1% vs. 8.7%); among white women (n=5354), lack of religious affiliation independently predicted multiple sexual partners, whereas among black women (n=2771), low or irregular church attendance did so.

- Wallace, J. M., and Forman, T. A. (1998). Religion's role in promoting health and reducing the risk among American youth. *Health Education and Behavior,* 25: 721–741. **Summary:** 5,000 students from 135 high schools across U.S. Importance of religion was inversely related to carrying a weapon to school, interpersonal violence, driving while drinking, riding while drinking, binge drinking, and marijuana use; but was positively related to seat belt use, better diet, exercise, and regular sleep patterns. Religious attendance also associated with fewer intentional and unintentional injury behaviors (except carrying a weapon), less substance use, and better health behaviors.

ACADEMIC AND POPULAR BOOKS

Academic

- *The Handbook of Religion and Health* by Harold G. Koenig, Michael E. McCullough, and David B. Larson (Oxford University Press, 2001). Comprehensive review of history, research, and discussion of religion and health. More than 700 pages, its thirty-five book chapters span mental and physical health, from well-being to depression to immune function, cancer, heart disease, stroke, chronic pain, disability, and others. Appendix lists twelve hundred separate scientific studies on religion and health that are reviewed and rated on 0–10 scale. Book ends with two thousand references and an extensive index for rapid topic identification. ($65)

- *The Link between Religion and Health: Psychoneuroimmunology and the Faith Factor* by Harold G. Koenig and Harvey Jay Cohen, eds. (Oxford University Press, 2002). Edited volume that examines the role of psychoneuroimmunology as an explanation for the link found between religion and physical health. Leaders in psychoneuroimmunology discuss their respective areas of research and how this research can help elucidate the relationship between religion and health. Reviews research on religious involvement, neuroendocrine and immune function, and explores further research needed to better understand these relationships. Fifteen chapters, approximately 300 pages. ($35)

- *Realized Religion: Research on the Relationship between Religion and Health* by Theodore J. Chamberlain and Christopher A. Hall (Templeton Foundation Press, 2000). Reviews research on the relationship between religion and health, and integrates research into an understanding of how and why this relationship exists. Easy to read and informative. Approximately 250 pages. ($30)

- *The Psychology of Religion and Coping* by Kenneth I. Pargament (Guilford Press, 1997). Reviews the literature on how religion is used when coping with crisis, including natural disasters (hurricanes, bombings, floods, etc.), health problems, and other major losses. Contains twelve chapters and more than 500 pages; probably the most comprehensive examination ever published on the theory, research, and practice of religious coping. ($50)

- *The Handbook of Religion and Mental Health* by Harold G. Koenig, ed. (Academic Press, 1998). Edited volume that examines the relationship between religion and stress, depression, anxiety, schizophrenia, and substance abuse. Explores how different religions (Catholic, Protestant, Mormon, Unity, Jewish, Buddhist, Hindu, Islam) understand mental health and how mental health practitioners should treat persons from different religious backgrounds; examines use of religion in psychotherapy; and discusses role of chaplain and role of community clergy in providing mental health. Twenty-five chapters, more than 400 pages. ($80)

- *Religion and the Clinical Practice of Psychology* by Edward P. Shafranske, ed. (American Psychological Association, 1996). Edited volume that focuses on the use of religion when working with religiously committed persons in therapy. Describes how to integrate religion from different traditions into clinical practice. Twenty-one chapters, more than 600 pages. ($60)

Popular (non-academic)

- *The Healing Connection* by Harold G. Koenig (Word, 2001). Quick reading, personal; examines some of the more recent research findings in a popular style. Directed primarily for the Christian reader. ($22)

- *God, Faith, and Health: Exploring the Spirituality-Healing Connection* by Jeffrey S. Levin (John Wiley and Sons, 2001). Quick reading, personal; reviews research findings on religion and health in a popular style. ($25)

- *The Healing Power of Faith* by Harold G. Koenig (Simon and Schuster, 2001). Quick reading; reviews research findings on religion and health in a popular style, illustrated with fascinating personal stories. ($25)

- *The Faith Factor* by Dale A. Matthews (Penguin, 1999). One of the first popular books to examine the relationship between traditional religious beliefs and practices and physical health, and to apply it to clinical practice. Numerous personal and heart-warming stories. ($14)

- *Is Religion Good for Your Health?* by Harold G. Koenig (Haworth Press, 1997). One of the first popular books to examine the relationship between traditional religious beliefs and practices and health. Has many graphs, figures, and facts, but no stories; good first book on topic. ($20)

WEBSITES, NEWSPAPERS, AND POPULAR MAGAZINES

Websites

- *Duke University's Center for the Study of Religion/Spirituality and Health.* Contains updated information on conferences, speakers, research reports, book reviews, and new two-year post-doctoral research fellowship program on religion and health. Provides a gateway to information on religion and health: www.geri.duke.edu.

- *International Center for the Integration of Health and Spirituality* (formerly NIHR). Contains updated information on conferences, speaker's bureau, research facts, summaries, and a newsletter. Director, David B. Larson, M.D., is a pioneer in the field: www.nihr.org

- *George Washington Institute for Spirituality and Health.* Focuses on medical education and gives out grants to medical schools to start courses on religion, spirituality, and medicine. Director, Christina Puchalski, M.D., is also an expert on spirituality in death and dying: www.gwish.org/index.htm

- *John Templeton Foundation.* Private foundation started by financial legend Sir John Templeton. The foundation sponsors research and conferences on spirituality, science, and health. Website provides information on grants, prizes, conferences, and other information in the area of religion and science: www.templeton.org

- *Mind-Body Medical Institute.* Started and directed by Herbert Benson, M.D., a widely known professor of medicine at Harvard Medical School. Focus is research and clinical practice in mind-body medicine. Sponsors the twice yearly *Spirituality and Healing in Medicine* continuing medical education conference of the Harvard Medical School: www.mbmi.org

Newspapers

- *Research News & Opportunities in Science and Theology.* A 36-page monthly newspaper distributed internationally with a circulation of about 30,000. Contains updated information on national news, research findings, national and regional meetings, education programs, books, discussions, organizations, and funding opportunities in the area of science, religion, and health (subscription price $10 for eleven issues/year). For more information and to sign up for a six-month free trial see website: www.researchnewsonline. org.

Popular Magazines

- *Spirituality and Health.* A quarterly 65-page magazine that focuses primarily on popular new age spirituality rather than on religion and health (subscription price $20 for four issues/year); for more information see website: www.spiritualityhealth.com

- *Science and Spirit.* Published six times per year, this popular magazine focuses primarily on religion and the physical sciences, although it does have occasional articles on health (subscription price $22 for six issues/year): www.science-spirit.org

NOTES

INTRODUCTION

1. King, D. (2000). *Faith, Spirituality, and Medicine: Toward the Making of the Healing Practitioner.* Binghamton, NY: Haworth Press.

2. Larson, D. B., Lu, F. G., Swyers, J. P. (1997). *Model Curriculum for Psychiatric Residency Training Programs: Religion and Spirituality in Clinical Practice.* Rockville, MD: National Institute for Healthcare Research.

3. Koenig, H. G., McCullough, M., Larson, D. B. (2001). *Handbook of Religion and Health.* New York: Oxford University Press.

4. Chibnall, J.T., Brooks, C.A. (2001). Religion in the clinic: the role of physician beliefs. *Southern Medical Journal, 94,* 374–379.

1. WHY INCLUDE SPIRITUALITY

1. Princeton Religion Research Center (1996). *Religion in America.* Princeton, NJ: The Gallup Poll.

2. Fitchett, G., Burton, L. A., and Sivan, A. B. (1997). The religious needs and resources of psychiatric patients. *Journal of Nervous and Mental Disease, 185,* 320–326.

3. Koenig, H. G. (2000). Religion, spirituality and medicine: Application to clinical practice. *Journal of the American Medical Association, 284,* 1708.

4. Rabin, B. (1999). *Stress, Immune Function, and Health: The Connection.* New York: Wiley.

5. Koenig, H. G., and Cohen, H. J. (2002). *The Link between Religion and Health: Psychoneuroimmunology and the Faith Factor.* New York: Oxford University Press.

6. Koenig, H. G. (1998). Religious beliefs and practices of hospitalized medically ill older adults. *International Journal of Geriatric Psychiatry, 13,* 213–224.

7. Princeton Religion Research Center (1982). *Religion in America.* Princeton, NJ: The Gallup Poll.

8. Saudia, T. L., Kinney, M. R., Brown, K. C., and Young-Ward, L. (1991). Health locus of control and helpfulness of prayer. *Heart and Lung, 20,* 60–65.

9. Cronan, T. A., Kaplan, R. M., Posner, L., Lumberg, E., and Kozin, F. (1989). Prevalence of the use of unconventional remedies for arthritis in a metropolitan community. *Arthritis and Rheumatism, 32,* 1604–1607.

10. Tix, A. P., and Frazier, P. A. (1997). The use of religious coping during stressful life events: Main effects, moderation, and mediation. *Journal of Consulting and Clinical Psychology, 66,* 411–422.

11. Stern, R. C., Canda, E. R., and Doershuk, C. F. (1992). Use of nonmedical treatment by cystic fibrosis patients. *Journal of Adolescent Health, 13,* 612–615.

12. Zaldivar, A., and Smolowitz, J. (1994). Perceptions of the importance placed on religion and folk medicine by non-Mexican-American Hispanic adults with diabetes. *The Diabetes Educator, 20,* 303–306.

13. Ell, K. O., Mantell, J. E., Hamovitch, M. B., and Nishimoto, R. H. (1989). Social support, sense of control, and coping among patients with breast, lung, or colorectal cancer. *Journal of Psychosocial Oncology, 7,* 63–89.

14. Roberts, J. A., Brown, D., Elkins, T., and Larson, D. B. (1997). Factors influencing views of patients with gynecologic cancer about end-of-life decisions. *American Journal of Obstetrics and Gynecology, 176,* 166–172.

15. Jenkins, R. A. (1995). Religion and HIV: Implications for research and intervention. *Journal of Social Issues, 51,* 131–144.

16. Abraido-Lanza, A. F., Guier, C., and Revenson, T. A. (1996). Coping and social support resources among Latinas with arthritis. *Arthritis Care and Research, 9*(6), 501–508.

17. Silber, T. J., Reilly, M. (1985). Spiritual and religious concerns of the hospitalized adolescent. *Adolescence, 20*(77), 217–224

18. Koenig, H. G., Weiner, D. K., Peterson, B. L., Meador, K. G., and Keefe F. J. (1998). Religious coping in institutionalized elderly patients. *International Journal of Psychiatry in Medicine, 27,* 365–376.

19. Wright, S. D., Pratt, C. C., and Schmall, V. L. (1985). Spiritual support for caregivers of dementia patients. *Journal of Religion and Health, 24,* 31–38.

20. Ehman, J, Ott, B., Short, T., Ciampa R., Hansen-Flaschen, J. (1999). Do patients want physicians to inquire about their spiritual or religious beliefs if they become gravely ill? *Archives of Internal Medicine, 159,* 1803–1806.

21. Kaldjian, L. C., Jekel, J. F., and Friedland, G. (1998). End-of-life decisions in HIV-positive patients: The role of spiritual beliefs. *AIDS, 12*(1), 103–107.

22. Koenig, H. G., McCullough, M. E., Larson, D. B. (2001). *Handbook of Religion and Health.* New York: Oxford University Press.

23. Koenig, H. G. (in press). An 83-year-old woman with chronic illness and strong religious beliefs (Clinical Crossroads). *Journal of the American Medical Association.*

24. Koenig, H. G., Cohen, H. J., Blazer, D. G., Pieper, C., and Meador, K. G., Shelp, F., Goli, V., and DiPasquale, R. (1992). Religious coping and depression in elderly hospitalized medically ill men. *American Journal of Psychiatry, 149,* 1693–1700.

25. Koenig, H. G., George, L. K., and Peterson, B. L. (1998). Religiosity and remission from depression in medically ill older patients. *American Journal of Psychiatry, 155,* 536–542.

26. Rabins, P. V., Fitting, M. D., Eastham, J., and Zabora, J. (1990). Emotional adaptation over time in care-givers for chronically ill elderly people. *Age and Ageing, 19,* 185–190.

27. Koenig et al. (2001).

28. Koenig et al. (2001).

29. Freud, S. (1962). Civilization and its discontents. In J. Strachey, (Ed. and Trans.), *Standard Edition of the Complete Psychological Works of Sigmund Freud.* London: Hogarth Press, 25. (Original work published in 1930).

30. Ellison, C. G., and George, L. K. (1994). Religious involvement, social ties, and social support in a southeastern community. *Journal for the Scientific Study of Religion, 33,* 46–61.

31. Koenig et al. (2001).

32. McEwen, B. S. (1998). Protective and damaging effects of stress mediators. *New England Journal of Medicine, 338,* 171–179.

33. Koenig, H. G., Cohen, H. J., George, L. K., Hays, J. C., Larson, D. B., Blazer, D. G. (1997). Attendance at religious services, interleukin-6, and other biological indicators of immune function in older adults. *International Journal of Psychiatry in Medicine, 27,* 233–250.

34. Woods, T. E., Antoni, M. H., Ironson, G. H., and Kling, D. W. (1999). Religiosity is associated with affective and immune status in symptomatic HIV-infected gay men. *Journal of Psychosomatic Research, 46,* 165–176.

35. Schaal, M. D., Sephton, S. E., Thoreson, C., Koopman, C., and Spiegel, D. (1998, August) *Religious Expression and Immune Competence in Women with Advanced Cancer.* Paper presented at the Meeting of the American Psychological Association, San Francisco, CA.

36. Koenig et al. (2001).

37. Colantonio, A., Kasl, S. V., and Ostfeld, A. M. (1992). Depressive symptoms and other psychosocial factors as predictors of stroke in elderly. *American Journal of Epidemiology, 136,* 884–894.

38. Goldbourt, U., Yaari, S., and Medalie, J. H. (1993). Factors predictive of long-term coronary heart disease mortality among 10,059 male Israeli civil servants and municipal employees. *Cardiology, 82,* 100–121.

39. Koenig et al. (2001).

40. Hummer, R., Rogers, R., Nam, C., and Ellison, C. G. (1999). Religious involvement and U.S. adult mortality. *Demography, 36,* 273–285.

41. Koenig H. G., Hays J. C., Larson D. B., George L. K., Cohen H. J., Mc-Cullough M., Meador K., Blazer D. G. (1999). Does religious attendance prolong survival?: A six-year follow-up study of 3,968 older adults. *Journal of Gerontology, Medical Sciences, 54A,* M370–M377

42. Strawbridge, W. J., Cohen, R. D., Shema, S. J., and Kaplan, G. A. (1997). Frequent attendance at religious services and mortality over 28 years. *American Journal of Public Health, 87,* 957–961.

43. Idler, E. L., and Kasl, S. V. (1997). Religion among disabled and nondisabled elderly persons, II: Attendance at religious services as a predictor of the course of disability. *Journal of Gerontology, 52B,* 306–316.

44. Koenig H. G., Larson D. B. (1998). Use of hospital services, church attendance, and religious affiliation. *Southern Medical Journal, 91,* 925–932

45. McNichol, T. (1996 April 5–7). The new faith in medicine. *USA Weekend,* p. 5.

46. Oyama, O., and Koenig, H. G. (1998). Religious beliefs and practices in family medicine. *Archives of Family Medicine, 7,* 431–435.

47. King, D. E., and Bushwick, B. (1994). Beliefs and attitudes of hospital inpatients about faith healing and prayer. *Journal of Family Practice, 39,* 349–352.

48. Kaldjian, L. C., Jekel, J. F., and Friedland, G. (1998). End-of-life decisions in HIV-positive patients: The role of spiritual beliefs. *AIDS, 12(1),* 103–107.

49. Ehman, J., Ott, B., Short, T., Ciampa R., Hansen-Flaschen, J. (1999). Do patients want physicians to inquire about their spiritual or religious beliefs if they become gravely ill? *Archives of Internal Medicine, 159,* 1803–1806.

50. Koenig, H. (2001). Religion, spirituality, and medicine: How are they related and what does it mean? *Mayo Clinic Proceedings, 76,* 1189–1191.

51. Taubes, T. (1998). "Healthy avenues of the mind": Psychological theory building and the influence of religion during the era of moral treatment. *American Journal of Psychiatry, 155,* 1001–1008.

2. *HOW* TO INCLUDE SPIRITUALITY

1. Koenig, H. G., Bearon, L., and Dayringer, R. (1989). Physician perspectives on the role of religion in the physician-older patient relationship. *Journal of Family Practice, 28,* 441–448.

2. Sloan, R. P., Bagiella, E., VandeCreek, L., Hover, M., Casalone, C., Hirsch, T.J., Hasan, Y., Kreger, R. (2000). Should physicians prescribe religious activities? *New England Journal of Medicine, 342,* 1913–1916.

3. Koenig, H. G., Bearon, L., and Dayringer, R. (1989). Physician perspectives on the role of religion in the physician-older patient relationship. *Journal of Family Practice, 28,* 441–448.

4. Koenig, H. G., Smiley, M., Gonzales, J. (1988). *Religion, Health, and Aging.* Westport, CT: Greenwood Press, 139.

5. King, D. E., and Bushwick, B. (1994). Beliefs and attitudes of hospital in-patients about faith healing and prayer. *Journal of Family Practice, 39,* 349–352.

6. Kaldjian, L. C., Jekel, J. F., and Friedland, G. (1998). End-of-life decisions in HIV-positive patients: The role of spiritual beliefs. *AIDS, 12*(1), 103–107.

7. Oyama, O., and Koenig, H. G. (1998). Religious beliefs and practices in family medicine. *Archives of Family Medicine, 7,* 431–435.

8. MacLean, C. D., Susi, B., Phifer, N., Schultz, L., Bynum, D., Franco, M., Klioze, A., Monroe, M., Garrett, J., Cykert, S. (in press). Religion and spirituality in the medical encounter: Results from a multi-center patient survey. *Journal of the American Medical Association.*

9. Yankelovich Parners, Inc., for *Time*/CNN, June 1996.

10. MacLean, et al. (2002).

11. Chibnall, J. T., and Brooks, C. A. (2001). Religion in the clinic: The role of physician beliefs. *Southern Medical Journal, 94,* 374–379.

12. Dagi, T. F. (1995). Prayer, piety, and professional propriety: Limits on religious expression in hospitals. *Journal of Clinical Ethics, 6,* 274–279.

13. Sloan, R. P., Bagiella, E., VandeCreek, L., Hover, M., Casalone, C., Hirsch, T. J., Hasan, Y., Kreger, R. (2000). Should physicians prescribe religious activities? *New England Journal of Medicine, 342,* 1913–1916.

14. Hale, W. E., Bennett, R. G. (2000). *Building Healthy Communities Through Medical-Religious Partnerships.* Baltimore, MD: Johns Hopkins University Press.

15. http://www.aoa.dhhs.gov/aoa/stats/AgePop2050.html.

16. Schneider, E. L. (1999). Aging in the third millennium. *Science, 283,* 796–797.

3. *WHEN* TO INCLUDE SPIRITUALITY

1. Cassem, N. H., Wishnie, H. A., Hackett, T. P. (1969). How coronary patients respond to last rites. *Postgraduate Medicine 45* (3), 147–152.

2. Benson, H., and Stark, M. (1996). *Timeless Healing: The Power and Biology of Belief.* New York: Simon and Schuster.

3. Feldstein, B. D. (2001). Toward meaning. *Journal of the American Medical Association, 286,* 1291–1292.

4. Dagi, T. F. (1995). Prayer, piety, and professional propriety: Limits on religious expression in hospitals. *Journal of Clinical Ethics, 6,* 274–279.

5. Post, S. G., Puchalski, C., Larson, D. (2000). Physicians and patient spirituality: professional boundaries, competency, and ethics. *Annals of Internal Medicine, 132,* 578–583.

4. WHAT MIGHT RESULT?

1. Most established traditional religious belief systems present a positive worldview, even some of those that on the surface don't appear to do so—such as fundamentalist systems that focus on sin, judgment, and retribution, and have rules that are harsh, rigid, and inflexible. These systems offer structure and clear guidelines on how to obtain relief through religious solutions and are usually quite sympathetic to sickness and adversity (although not always).

2. Osler, W. (1910). The faith that heals. *The British Medical Journal,* 1470–1472.

3. Safran, D. G., Taira, D. A., Rogers, W. H., Kosinski, M., Ware, J. E., Tarlov, A.R. (1998). Linking primary care performance to outcomes of care. *Journal of Family Practice, 47*(3), 213–220.

4. Thom, D. H., Ribisl K. M., Stewart A. L., Luke D. A. (1999). Further validation and reliability testing of the Trust in Physician Scale. The Stanford Trust Study Physicians. *Medical Care, 37*(5), 510–517.

5. Koenig, H. G. et al. (2001). Disease prevention, disease detection, and treatment compliance, *Handbook of Religion and Health* (pp. 397–408).

6. Koenig, H. G., Shelp, F., Goli, V., Cohen, H. J., Blazer, D. G. (1989). Survival and healthcare utilization in elderly medical inpatients with major depression. *Journal of the American Geriatrics Society, 37,* 599–606.

7. Kiecolt-Glaser, J. K., Marucha, P. T., Malarkey, W. B., Mercado, A. M., and Glaser, R. (1996). Slowing of wound healing by psychological stress. *Lancet, 346*(8984), 1194–1196.

8. Benson, H., and Stark, M. (1996). *Timeless Healing: The Power and Biology of Belief.* New York: Simon and Schuster.

5. BOUNDARIES AND BARRIERS

1. Pelligrino, E. (1979). Toward a reconstruction of medical morality: The primacy of the act of profession and the fact of illness. *Journal of Medicine and Philosophy, 4,* 32–56.

2. Forster, J. (2000, January 10). Retake your Hippocratic oath. *Medical Economics.*

3. Butler, A. M. (1968). Hippocratic oath, 1968. *New England Journal of Medicine, 278,* 48–49.

4. Translated by Harry Friedenwald, *Bulletin of the Johns Hopkins Hospital, 28,* 260–261, (1917).

5. Spero, M. H. (1981). Countertransference in religious therapists of religious patients. *American Journal of Psychotherapy, 35,* 565–575.

6. Koenig, H. G., Hover, M., Bearon, L. B., Travis, J.L. (1991). Religious perspectives of doctors, nurses, patients and families: Some interesting differences. *Journal of Pastoral Care, 45,* 254–267.

7. Ellis, M. R., Vinson, D. C., Ewigman, B. (1999). Addressing spiritual concerns of patients: Family physicians' attitudes and practices. *Journal of Family Practice, 48,* 105–109.

8. Chibnall, J. T., and Brooks, C. A. (2001). Religion in the clinic: The role of physician beliefs. *Southern Medical Journal, 94,* 374–379.

9. Chalfant, H. P., Heller , P. L., Roberts, A., Briones, D., Aquirre-Hochbaum, S., Farr, W. (1990). The clergy as a resource for those encountering psychological distress. *Review of Religious Research, 31,* 305–313.

10. Larson, D. B., Hohmann, A. A., Kessler, L. G., Meador, K. G., Boyd, J. H., and McSherry, E. (1988). The couch and the cloth: The need for linkage. *Hospital and Community Psychiatry, 39,* 1064–1069.

11. Chibnall and Brooks (2001).

12. Koenig, H. G., Bearon, L., and Dayringer, R. (1989). Physician perspectives on the role of religion in the physician-older patient relationship. *Journal of Family Practice, 28,* 441–448.

13. Koenig et al., (1989).

14 . Maugans, T. A., Wadland, W. C. (1991). Religion and family medicine: A survey of physicians and patients. *Journal of Family Practice, 32,* 210–213.

6. WHEN RELIGION IS HARMFUL

1. Sloan, R. P., Bagiella, E.,and Powell, T. (1999). Religion, spirituality, and medicine. *The Lancet, 353,* 664–667.

2. Sloan, R. P., Bagiella, E., VandeCreek, L., Hover, M., Casalone, C., Hirsch, T.J., Hasan, Y., Kreger, R. (2000). Should physicians prescribe religious activities? *New England Journal of Medicine, 342,* 1913–1916.

3. Spence, C., Danielson, T. S., and Kaunitz, W. M. (1984, March). The Faith Assembly: A study of perinatal and maternal mortality. *Indiana Medicine,* pp. 180–183.

4. Conyn–Van Spaendonck, M. A., de Melker, H. E., Abbink, F., Elzinga–Gholizadea, N., Kimman, T. G., van Loon, T. (2001). Immunity to poliomyelitis in the Netherlands. *American Journal of Epidemiology, 153*(3), 207–214.

5. *Morbidity and Mortality Weekly Report* (1991). Outbreaks of rubella among the Amish—United States, 1991. *Morbidity and Mortality Weekly Report, 40*(16), 264–265.

6. Etkind, P., Lett, S. M., MacDonald, P. D., Silva, E., and Peppe, J. (1992). Pertussis outbreaks in groups claiming religious exemptions to vaccinations. *American Journal of Diseases of Children, 146,* 173–176.

7. Rodgers, D. V., Gindler, J. S., Atkinson, W. L., and Markowitz, L. E. (1993). High attack rates and case fatality during a measles outbreak in groups with religious exemption to vaccination. *Pediatric Infectious Disease Journal, 12,* 288–292.

8. Coakley, D. V., and McKenna, G. W. (1986, February 22). Safety of faith healing. *Lancet,* p. 444.

9. Smith, D. M. (1986, March 15). Safety of faith healing. *Lancet,* p. 621.

10. Asser, S., and Swan R. (1998). Child fatalities from religion-motivated medical neglect. *Pediatrics, 101,* 625–629.

11. Koenig, H. G., McCullough, M. E., Larson, D. B. (2001). *Handbook of Religion and Health.* New York: Oxford University Press, 63–71.

12. Pargament, K. I., Koenig, H. G., Tarakeshwar, N., Hahn, J. (2001). Religious struggle as a predictor of mortality among medically ill elderly patients: A two-year longitudinal study. *Archives of Internal Medicine, 161,* 1881–1885.

13. Sloan et al.(1999), 666.

14. Pargament et al. (2001).

7. RESOURCES

1. Kuhn, C. C. (1988). A spiritual inventory of the medically ill patient. *Psychiatric Medicine, 6,* 87–100.

2. Matthews, D. A., and Clark, C. (1998). *The Faith Factor.* New York: Viking.

3. Matthews, D. A., McCullough, M. E., Larson, D. B., Koenig, H. G., Swyers, J. P., Milano, M. G. (1998). Religious commitment and health status: A review of the research and implications for family medicine. *Archives of Family Medicine 7,* 118–124.

4. Puchalski, C. M., Romer, A. L. (2000). Taking a spiritual history allows clinicians to understand patients more fully. *Journal of Palliative Medicine, 3,* 129–137.

5. Maugans, T. A. (1996). The SPIRITual history. *Archives of Family Medicine, 5,* 11–16.

6. Anandarajah, G., Hight, E. (2001). Spirituality and medical practice: Using the HOPE questions as a practical tool for spiritual assessment. *American Family Physician, 63*(1), 81–88.

7. Lo, B., Quill, T., Tulsky, J. (1999). Discussing palliative care with patients. *Annals of Internal Medicine, 130,* 744–749.

INDEX